two
old
broads

two old broads

Stuff You Need to Know That You Didn't Know *You Needed to Know*

M. E. HECHT, MD
and Whoopi Goldberg

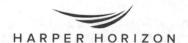

HARPER HORIZON

Two Old Broads

© 2022 Whoopi Goldberg and M. E. Hecht, MD

All rights reserved. No portion of this book may be reproduced, stored in a retrieval system, or transmitted in any form or by any means—electronic, mechanical, photocopy, recording, scanning, or other—except for brief quotations in critical reviews or articles, without the prior written permission of the publisher.

Published by Harper Horizon, an imprint of HarperCollins Focus LLC.

Book design by Aubrey Khan, Neuwirth & Associates, Inc.
Stethoscope icon by Rokhman Kharis from Noun Project.com
Glasses icon by John Caserta from NounProject.com

Any internet addresses, phone numbers, or company or product information printed in this book are offered as a resource and are not intended in any way to be or to imply an endorsement by Harper Horizon, nor does Harper Horizon vouch for the existence, content, or services of these sites, phone numbers, companies, or products beyond the life of this book.

ISBN 978-0-7852-4165-2 (Ebook)
ISBN 978-0-7852-4164-5 (HC)
ISBN 978-1-4003-3515-2 (B&N edition)

Library of Congress Control Number: 2022934024

Printed in the United States of America
22 23 24 25 26 LSC 10 9 8 7 6 5 4 3 2 1

To my sine qua non, D.
There are no words; you already know them.

Contents

Dating (Another Take) *39*

Sex Over Sixty? *45*

Is There Life After Jimmy Choo? *49*

Girdles *53*

Excursions *57*

PART THREE
Broad Bones

The Aches and Pains Hour *63*

Patients as Junior Partners *65*

Four Ears Plus One Notepad Equals a Winner! *69*

A Visit to the Doctor: Never a One-Way Street *71*

Fear of Surgery from a Surgeon's Point of View *77*

Medical Second Opinions *81*

Getting Choosy *85*

Fear of Anesthesia *89*

Don't Get Ripped *91*

You and Your Ears *97*

Dental Phobia *101*

PART FOUR
Broad Well-Being

How to Train Your Keeper *109*

Inactivity: The Enemy *113*

Don't Get Out of Bed So Soon *117*

Senior Skin Care *123*

Sports and Physical Activity *127*

Living in the Past *133*

The Time I Ignored My Own Advice *135*

Contents

Introduction . . . . *xiii*

PART ONE
Broad Mentality

———

Our Broad Experience *3*
You Are Not a Number *5*
Eliminate the Negative! *9*
Your Marvelous Machine *11*
It's Been a Good Long While *15*
Wisdom *19*
You're a Guru *21*

PART TWO
Broad Life

———

O Tempora, O Mores
    (Oh the Times, Oh the Customs)—Cicero *25*
Friendship Through the Ages *29*
Dress Like a Broad *33*
Dating (An Entirely Different Subject) *37*

We dedicate this book
with care and respect
to all Old Broads,
of any color, creed, or disposition,
whenever and wherever they abide.
They've survived the past, handled the present,
and so, by example,
offer hope to generations yet to come.

Contents

After the Fall *139*

Medications: Take Full Control *143*

Self-Examination (Yes, I Do Mean Yours!) *151*

PART FIVE
Broad Shoulders

Am I Losing My Mind? *159*

Nodding Off *163*

An Approach to Your Will *169*

Let's Talk About Attrition *173*

Breaking Medical News *177*

Crotchety with Charm *183*

PART SIX
Broad Insights

Lists Are Your Friends *187*

A Morning Prayer *189*

Who Are You Calling Eccentric? *191*

The Sunday Comics *195*

Grow Old or Grow Up? *197*

Battle Hymn of the Republic *201*

An Evening Prayer *203*

Vale Dicta (Last Words) *205*

Broad Encore *207*

Epilogue: In Memory of M. E. Hecht, MD *209*

Acknowledgments *211*

Index *213*

About the Authors *221*

Introduction

They say, "Sixty is the new forty." And our response is:
Why can't we treat sixty as sixty and be proud of it?
WHOOPI GOLDBERG AND DR. M. E. HECHT

Forget putting those of us over sixty "on a shelf." Forget the terms *old lady, elder, over the hill, granny,* and *geriatric.* We're with Aretha Franklin—it's time we Broads got some *r-e-s-p-e-c-t.*

Here, we (Whoopi Goldberg and close friend Dr. M. E. Hecht) share stories and commentary about stuff you didn't know you need to know as we age.

Two Old Broads is a funny and informative book that speaks directly to women ages sixty plus and those of you who have not yet attained the advantage. We invite you all to laugh and feel proud as we offer thoughts and insider information on how to navigate some of the complex issues of this time in life—with no apologies.

A book like this is just what the doctor ordered. With one of us (Whoopi) writing as a woman in her sixties and one of us (Dr. Hecht) writing as a woman in her nineties, we dish truths and tales, each sharing our Broad experiences that show wisdom, spirit, intelligence, humor, sensibility, and most importantly, our collective, extraordinary "Broadness."

A NOTE FROM M. E. HECHT (DR. H)

Whoopi and I have spent many holidays together. The last time we were together was Christmas Day 2019, and when most of our party had gone home, we went on talking into the small hours as old friends do. Aging was a large part of our conversation, and that's where we hatched the idea for *Two Old Broads*.

Whoopi Goldberg (Whoop to me) is a household name, but I'm not sure many of you know much about this Broad: me, Dr. M. E. Hecht. So, please, let me introduce myself.

I was born in 1929 in Baltimore, Maryland, home of the best oysters and steamed crabs and the Orioles. My family was in the department store business, and, due to the smarts of my grandfather, we survived and prospered during the difficult 1930s.

My father was just young enough to be drafted for WWII, and he was assigned to the US Army Quartermaster Corps in Savannah, Georgia. I was shipped off to a girls' boarding school, the Shipley School in Bryn Mawr, Pennsylvania. There, I received top-level schooling focused on English lit, history, and various languages.

After four years, I left Pennsylvania to return to my hometown, Baltimore, and got into off-off-off-Broadway (otherwise identifiable as local theater)—at least the technical side of it (lighting, stage management, stage design, etc.). Then I moved to New York City, where, in between working on real off-Broadway productions, I earned a BA from New York University. My summers were spent with what was then a flourishing summer theater group. To give you a sense of how well attended and high caliber these performances were, I'm going to drop a few names of the actors I worked with. Those of you over age sixty will glom these: Cesar Romero, Bea Lillie, Madge Evans, Nigel Bruce, and Gloria Vanderbilt.

Then followed an MA from Yale University's theatrical school. Again, I was still focused on the technical aspect of theater. This led to several years working on Broadway as an associate producer with Alex Cohen.

One day, at the age of thirty-two, I decided to change course and go to medical school for the same apocryphal reason people give when they decide to climb Mount Everest: because it was there.

I graduated in 1966 and went into the practice of orthopedics. As time went by, I had the pleasure of two innovative experiences. In 1982, I founded a second-surgical-opinion group for patients considering elective (versus emergency) surgery. I later headed up one of the early established ambulatory surgeries for Mother Cabrini Hospital in NYC.

Upon retirement from the active practice of orthopedic surgery in the 1990s, I started to write. In the beginning, I wrote medical articles and books for patients; later I wrote fiction. If I had to summarize my career, I think you might agree that it could be described as "checkered." I've been around the block three times or so.

Back when I was coming into my Broad years, people didn't talk about aging. Numbers were all-important—if you were a certain age, people thought they knew all they needed to know about you. Both Whoopi and I hope that as you read the pieces herein, you'll find that numbers—in and of themselves—are pointless. It's what you know, think, share, and imagine that make a really great Old Broad.

Whoopi, as I'm sure you know, has had an even more varied and successful career—not to mention her life experiences. We both hope that sharing about the things we've learned or done will strike you as helpful, even practical, but above all that you'll appreciate our light-handed insights here in *Two Old Broads*.

A WORD FROM WHOOPI

When Dr. Hecht and I first talked about this book, there was no COVID-19, there was no quarantining in place, kids went to school, people were cranky, you-know-who was still in the White House, and our mouths were just starting to drop at the audaciousness of politicians.

Well, now it's been nearly two years since the pandemic started in the US, and we're seeing the craziest of crazy things happen and left wondering why it's so nuts right now. If you're over fifty, you're probably trying to figure out what the eff is going on. Because all of the things that your folks told you when you were younger (e.g., don't lie, don't cheat, or else you will be scorned) seem to be gone.

And I think a lot of our crotchetiness is because it feels like none of those things were true in the first place. People lie, and nobody seems to be upset about it. Nobody is saying, "Hey, I'm scorning you. I don't like a liar because I can't trust you." Or how about cheating. Nowadays, when people cheat on a test or plagiarize, there seems to be no consequence. And I think this bothers people, yet they don't know what to do. So they just suck it up, keep it in their stomachs, and walk around stoically.

Now put on top of that the seeming disappearance of common sense. Who would have thought wearing a mask or not wearing a mask would have people close to throwing blows? I mean, if you woke up in a surgical room and none of your doctors or nurses were wearing a mask, I think you'd be freaking out. I know I would. Because you know they wear those masks as protection from whatever is in that room. You can sterilize that room all you want, but little bitty contaminants can get in. Doctors and nurses have to wear masks to protect themselves, each other, and their patients—so I don't understand why, "Hey, can you wear a mask because it protects me and you?" have become fighting words.

Maybe my crotchety, "Old Broad" perspective developed just because I've gotten older; who can say. Regardless, a lot of what you're gonna read in this book, at least from me, was written through a COVID-19 lens. But there's another important perspective you'll be getting too.

PART ONE
Broad Mentality

I am where I am because I believe in all possibilities.
WHOOPI GOLDBERG

———

OUR BROAD EXPERIENCE

YOU ARE NOT A NUMBER

ELIMINATE THE NEGATIVE!

YOUR MARVELOUS MACHINE

IT'S BEEN A GOOD LONG WHILE

WISDOM

YOU'RE A GURU

Our Broad Experience

DR. H AND WHOOPI

s there something reasonably pleasing and apropos that we want to call ourselves as women over sixty? It seems everyone else wants to call us "old ladies." This is such BS. Men get the gravitas of becoming "distinguished" and "well-seasoned" with age, while, somehow, women become invisible. But maybe it's us; maybe we accommodate or even permit the attitude. Which is a shame because, if the past reveals one thing, it's that the world needs more Broads.

We're now Experienced Broads. Experience makes us think of a journey—and it's a journey all of us are on. But you'd be surprised how offended some people still get about calling a female "Broad." In the movie business, Broads like Mae West were very popular in the 1930s, but today they are a rare breed. West tossed out double entendres in a saucy tone that left no room for misinterpretation, but that's not the only way she showed up as a Broad. A Broad knows her purpose and owns her presence. Think: Rosa Parks, Josephine Baker, Katharine Hepburn, Ruth Bader Ginsburg, and Michelle Obama. Broads, all.

It is our hope that you share the Broad experience and pass it along or offer some of your hard-earned wisdom to your younger near and dear. We know that they need it.

So . . . is a Broad:

Feisty? You bet.

Fun? You bet.

Gutsy? You bet.

Incisive? You bet.

Original? You bet.

Even off color? You bet.

Call me a Broad? Please!

Call *you* a Broad? Consider this your invitation to join the club!

You Are Not a Number

DR. H

Even as your body is telling on you, don't dream of interjecting into a verbal exchange—whether in person, on the phone, or by any other means—the words: "I'm _____ years old." It doesn't matter if that age is sixty-five, seventy-five, eighty-five, or even ninety-five. As a point of interest, this should be irrelevant to anyone hearing those words, with the exception of medical personnel and census workers.

When you lead a sentence with your age, it gives listeners tacit permission to presume, *She's too old to get it,* and exclude you from many subjects—which is the last thing you should want.

How dare we let a number become of such interest, importance, or legitimacy. It's a large, miserable mistake to use age as an excuse of any kind.

BE PRESENT AND PROUD

The most interesting things about you at any age, and especially as you arrive at your senior years, are who you are, what you've done, and what you've achieved. It's your job to keep this perspective always in your mind and to develop conversations around your experiences that are worth discussing with others.

Don't be afraid to talk about what you are doing, a skill or talent you possess, or something new you are learning.

For instance, are you into knitting? Ask someone if they want a sweater.

Are you into ikebana? It's the Japanese flower arrangement that represents the balance of sun, moon, and earth. Tell someone about it.

Do you do sudoku or the daily newspaper crossword? Ask for tips.

What's your *Jeopardy!* score compared to the panel member each session? Share that!

The ears around you will listen up when you engage them in a new topic. If, for example, you're working on a crossword puzzle, say something like, "I got to twenty-seven down, and I'm stuck." Nine out of ten times, the person you are with will come to your side, look at the puzzle, and say, "Try this," or "Darned if I know." In any case, you'll have engaged in a meeting of equals.

Or, if you're sitting at the dining table with your family, make an inquiry to the person who cooked the meal, such as, "What did you put in the cake/soup/stew to make it so delicious?" You can bet a one-to-one conversation will develop, and this is the kind of exchange you should always try for as a senior. Start initiating them!

No matter how ironic this seems, you must earn your wings by making relevant comments or contributions to combat age exclusion. Even if you're in an assisted living facility, the other residents shouldn't find your number of much interest. So just plain knock it out of conversations!

When you're asked directly to share the number of years you've lived on this planet, you may answer simply, but then immediately move on to focus the conversation on an unrelated subject. For example: "Thanks for asking. I've gotten to be eighty-five. By the way, what did you think of the Academy Awards this year (or the Academy of Country Music Awards or state elections)?"

You get the point. Gears will shift, not to mention interest.

So, no more expiations of the number of years you've been around. Move on to what interests you about *current* happenings or what you're doing now. Better still, talk about what your hearer is interested in.

Remember, your age is not what matters. What matters about you is what you're doing, who you're trying to be today, and what your goals or hopes are for the future. Yes, the future. Dare to discuss it.

But if you feel like you're fated to sit at the bottom of the conversational table, there are a couple of things I suggest:

1. If it's something critical, whoever is saying it will find a way to convey it to you.
2. Nearly invisible hearing aids are now easily available. Many are covered by Medicare. They don't restore complete hearing, but I'd say at least two-thirds to three-fourths (not too shabby).

Final thought: unless someone specifically asks you to enumerate your aches, activity limitations, or physical or social problems, *keep them to yourself.* In the end, those things are only important to you!

By now it should be proven beyond a doubt: you are *not* a number.

Eliminate the Negative!

WHOOPI

∞

Well, the only way to really eliminate the negative in life is, at five o'clock each evening, to put your phone away, keep the news turned off, and take a walk. On this walk just think about the good stuff. *So far so good. I made it through this much of the day. I'd like to make it through some more.* Think about the things you like, the things that make you happy.

There's enough time—there's twenty-four hours for goodness' sake—for you to get all angry at whoever or whatever, but you gotta take at least half an hour to just be ridiculous inside your own mind. Be as ridiculous as you want to be.

Listen, there is enough stress to last you day in and day out, so why not say, "You know what? I'm going to fart every twenty feet I go." Say it in your head. And if it makes you laugh, that's a good thing. You gotta find things that will make you chuckle, just for yourself. Nobody else has to get the joke. Most people don't even get other people's jokes, unless they're professionally written.

Let me tell you my favorite clean joke. You can tell it to yourself: A man is walking down the beach, and he looks over and sees an oyster and a lobster making love. He thinks, *Well I've never seen that before.* And he watches. And when they're done, the lobster drags himself off into the water, and the man walks over to the oyster and says, "Excuse me, miss."

"Yes?" she says in a high-pitched voice.

"Did I just see you making love to a lobster?" he says.

"Oh yes," she says. "Yes, you did. Yes, you did."

"Well, what's that like?" he says.

And she says, "Well, he put one claw here, and another claw here, and—" she gasps. "*My pearls!*"

Make yourself laugh. End of joke.

DR. H'S TWO CENTS

This advice is an absolute must for those entering their seventies and eighties. There was a popular singer whose career spanned from the 1930s well into the millennium. He appeared with Grace Kelly and Frank Sinatra in a movie called *High Society.* Many of you will remember Bing Crosby.

Well, in addition to being a talented golfer, he popularized a song that should become a second national anthem: "Ac-Cent-**Tchu**-Ate the Positive." You can still download this classic or listen to it on YouTube. It's still highly relevant today.

As an aside, no, I never played golf with Bing Crosby, who was a very low handicap amateur (as was Bob Hope). But Ed Sullivan and I played many times with Althea Gibson (US Open tennis champ), who hit the ball farther than most men.

Your Marvelous Machine

DR. H

With over thirty years of medical knowledge and expertise working with patients, I am continually amazed by what I believe is the most sophisticated organism on earth, a scientific marvel: the human body, our marvelous machine!

I don't know whether you've thought about it, but your body is a machine. Made of muscles, bones, a few organs, and yes, even a brain. But it's as absolutely unique as your fingerprints. (Did you know that even identical twins do not have the same fingerprints? That's because fingerprints are formed completely independently— by touching your surroundings while in the womb.) The human body is so sophisticated and multiproductive that even the most advanced AI, algorithms, and scientists can't begin to duplicate it.

I was first exposed to the intricate nature of the human body in medical school. No one really asks orthopedists why they went into the specialty. But for me it was several reasons, one of which was because the human body has always reminded me of an automobile.

Let's say you've decided to buy an automobile (nothing as complicated as the space shuttle or even the USS *New Hampshire*).

This is just a car that you will use at your leisure or for necessary transportation. What's involved? What is the all-in investment in this automobile?

In year one you'll spend money on:

1. The purchase price (thousands!)
2. Taxes on this purchase
3. Insurance
4. Gas/electric
5. Commitment to the 30/60/90 schedule, meaning certain items need to be inspected, changed, or replaced at thirty thousand, sixty thousand, and ninety thousand miles

In year two the cost looks like:

1. Yearly major servicing and maintenance
2. Gas/electric
3. Periodic washing and cleaning (or time and effort to do so on your own when you'd rather be shopping or watching a critical football or basketball game)
4. Insurance renewal (likely increased if you've had a fender bender)
5. Some part replacements and software updates

In years three, four, five, and six, in addition to having a car with a much less shiny appearance, dings, and aged interiors, you'll have to contend with:

1. Extensive and expensive part replacements (like tires, brakes, etc.)
2. All the additional expenses of year two

Then, somewhen in the next decade, you'll have to consider: Do you still have the same gas guzzler? Do people honk and hold their noses as they pass you? Are you sure the old dear will start up on a cold winter's morning? Even knowing you may be a parsimonious soul, does your family finally say, "Enough! The time has come to shell out for new transportation"? If yes, you'll be back to the cost and bother of year one.

Automobiles are complicated systems with many interconnected parts that perform specialized chores—much like the human body. The engine is the heart; it makes the machine run. The safety devices are the car's eyes and ears. And the main part of the car is its software, like the human brain. When we are ill, physicians look up our medical histories to understand our prior health and usually suggest tests to understand what may be wrong. With cars, mechanics use their software to understand the car's previous state and assess what may be wrong.

At this point, it must be observed that every machine, whether mechanical or human, exists with frailties that need to be dealt with in individual ways. But unlike the relatively short life expectancy of cars, today's medical care and knowledge have advanced to the point where living to seventy, eighty, or even ninety years of age is not remarkable. True, your human machine may need more attention and care at this point—perhaps even some optional replacements—but you can't simply trade it in for a newer model. Instead, you should reward it for all its years of loyal service by treating it well!

Our bodies and minds are capable of growth, adaptation, creativity, and mobility that age does not have to limit. We really can actively maintain our marvelous machines so they will go a distance beyond now—and perhaps beyond what we've ever dreamed.

It's Been a Good
Long While

DR. H

For those of you who are New Old Broads—or maybe those who aren't quite as old of Broads as I am—let's talk about this concept of time. Time happens to all of us (like molasses when you're a child, like a runaway train when you pass forty), but when you become a Broad, you have more control over the ways in which you do or think or spend it.

Here's what I mean. When I was young, as perhaps was true for many of you, too, time was an endless endurance of events over which I had no control whatsoever. From the moment I rose until I was asleep, time was both parsed and defined for me. Meals, bathing, dressing, and naps were ironclad events that happened, requiring my presence, at exact times. Time was a personal imposition, even more a frustration, in those early years.

As I grew a little older, time became more defined by school schedules, birthday parties, or vacations that began to fit a certain yearly pattern. Their rhythm and formality were helpful.

In the next stage of growth, time became more interesting because of the physical changes in my body that accompanied the years. Sex, sports, and anatomic changes became a function of time. This is the phase of life when many of us want more and more time in which to do things!

Young adulthood, with academic pursuits and employment, became entirely a matter of set schedules. In this phase, events occurred primarily at the convenience of other people or institutions.

And call it as it lies, the middle years, i.e., more or less forty to sixty, are a mess, full of things like divorce, sleepless nights, menopause brain, fad diets, and the awareness that youth is long gone and will not return. Time becomes a matter of such things as inappropriate clothing to name but a few mischances that inhabit for many these potentially miserable years, or as someone once said, too young to be old and too old to be young. Forty to sixty is also the time of knowing who you are and seeing your kids leave the nest . . . and not necessarily with a thank you.

However, with the arrival of our sixties and seventies, time becomes a much more complex event. Sometimes it's a matter of contemplation, sometimes it moves at our behest, sometimes it is dictated by the convenience of others. Regardless, I found that, for me, it gained a certain fluidity during these years.

But sometimes, during this phase, we are left wondering, *When and how did I get here?* Perhaps for the first time, the question comes as a matter for serious speculation, and it may even bring about some degree of fear. This is when time becomes largely defined by our physical bodies—arthritis, hypertension, and coronary problems, among others that can show up.

However, in the quiet of late night, on my way to bed and sleep, I often review the chances life has offered me, those taken and those not. It makes for an interesting bedtime rehearsal. One piece of advice that I lean on, which may be good for you too: be gentle on the parts that were good or interesting or positive, and let the rest go absent with sleep.

Perhaps another way of thinking about time as an Old Broad is that now, the intervals between sleep and wake, between societal or family-type events—even medical appointments—define the passage of time. Yet, simultaneously, we Broads cannot afford to wake with the notion of, "What shall I do today to make time pass?" Such thinking is only marginally better than taking an over-large sleeping draught or even the traditional arsenic-laced double shot of booze. Instead, I suggest listing for yourself all the things you find favorable or interesting or tasty or intriguing or mystifying or even funny. And arrange to do them!

Schedule each day with a minimum of three of those activities or ideas—things that are just for you. And make sure they're done with both savor and recognition. Do this in your timing and nobody else's.

One of the things I have control over is the menu for the day. Being a foodie, I always include three favorites so that if one gets crossed off the list, I can still have the other two!

As an elderly writer with short-term memory problems, each night I write down the things that should be done the next day, including any preparation these things may require for complete execution. If I don't write them down, they are likely to be wiped from my memory by morning. I have little notepads all over the house. I even have a pen that lights up just the pad at night; one of the really great stocking stuffers I've received over these many years!

I've also found the benefit in taking time just before sleep to recall fun, rewarding, helpful, and even bizarre times, people, and holidays from my past. Doing so is a way to re-enjoy them.

There's no promise that anything I suggest here will slow or prevent the passage of unwanted time.

But if you feel like you are missing out on the time you have left, remember: much of what you may have missed is not life and death, not even earthshaking, so take in what you can, pursue things that are interesting, new, or educational, and always find new ways to laugh!

Wisdom

DR. H

The word—no, the concept of—wisdom has a kind of biblical ring to it. And yet it must be applied to our daily thoughts, actions, and responsibilities, especially when we attain our seniority or Broadness.

To put it less formally, by the time we arrive at our senior years, we better damn well have achieved smarts, through experience and some formal learning.

In our early years, our judgment is often clouded by our emotions, so we devote our energy to action more than thought. Then we have to buckle down and get serious when it comes to life, our kids, their kids, and the everyday demands of being an adult. In other words, if we are to make serious mistakes, they are best confined to, let's say, the first thirty- or fortyish years of our lives.

For example, when many of us arrive at our teenage years and even beyond, we feel that the counsel, advice, and cautions of our parents have no place or relevance. Their hazards, achievements, modes of communication, and even lessons about historical events are seemingly not germane to our generation or to us as individuals. I, for one, felt in my formative years that I could self-invent as the need or situation arrived, and counsel was of small meaning. Especially that of my parents.

How wrong I was!

I have now lived for over ninety years, and it turns out that much of what my mother had to say was—and remains—entirely relevant to my present station, condition, and circumstances.

You can gift your near and dear (especially the younger generation) with your wisdom. You may have to adjust the language you use by sprinkling in some digital mentions, hip phrases, or references to popular phone apps, but speak from the experience you've gained. No matter the subject, your history validates what you have to say as nothing else can.

Turning to a more domestic arena, your wisdom (or, if you prefer the shorter word, "smarts") can help your juniors with parenting. You can share the history of what you did right as well as some unfortunate missteps or approaches to be avoided. Many of the problems you faced and even some parenting terms have not changed. So your experience, laced as it is with wisdom, has a chance of being recognized, valued, and even followed!

Your grandchildren, especially if curious—or, better still, intelligent—may even ask about your life experiences as they seek help navigating the passage through any age. The actual age difference somehow gives them the good sense to recognize that the world goes round and round on an off tilt, but the dawn rises, and the sun sets. In one part of the world or another, dusk and dawn always arrive. The circumstances of what they must face may change, but the heart of the growing-up experience translates!

I am wise, I am senior, and I can pass along wisdom.

You're a Guru

DR. H

In many cultures around the world, seniors are highly treasured, even honored. It comes as a part of becoming an elder. In our country, it seems you need to work to earn honor and respect. To which we clever Old Broads say, "If so, so be it."

We've put in the work through years of experiences, nuts, mishaps, and successes. Winning and, yes, losing can be informative as hell. Now is the time to use everything life has, one way or another, bestowed.

Open your mouth and tell others about your life. The sign over your desk might not read "Guru," but as an experienced Old Broad, this is what you've become. History is a unique, irreplaceable, often unforgiving teacher about which there is a cogent saying: "He who forgets history is doomed to repeat it"! You, with a more panoramic view of events than your juniors, may clearly recognize this truth. You really should be obligated to iterate the history lessons you've learned.

For example, you may either have experienced or know about the hardship created by the Dust Bowl of the 1930s and how it was largely the result of drought plus inadvisable agricultural practices.

Now think of today's parallel: the current use of pesticides that have decimated the honeybee population that is so critical in pollinating crop plants and fruit trees, not to mention their venom's possible use as a cancer inductive in humans. Another parallel is the extremes of weather and ensuing weather disasters most likely induced by climate change.

The name or terms of what they must face may change, but the heart of the experience translates!

PART TWO
Broad Life

Normal is just a cycle on the washing machine.
WHOOPI GOLDBERG

———

O TEMPORA, O MORES (OH THE TIMES,
OH THE CUSTOMS)—CICERO

FRIENDSHIP THROUGH THE AGES

DRESS LIKE A BROAD

DATING (AN ENTIRELY DIFFERENT SUBJECT)

DATING (ANOTHER TAKE)

SEX OVER SIXTY?

IS THERE LIFE AFTER JIMMY CHOO?

GIRDLES

EXCURSIONS

O Tempora, O Mores (Oh the Times, Oh the Customs)—Cicero

DR. H

A t the respective ages that Whoop and I are now, finding new friends can be a challenge. As time goes on, it's inescapable not to have lost—and, unfortunately, continue to lose—friends. Our social circles begin to shrink, friendly acquaintances disappear (especially after the pandemic). Because of Whoop's extensive work on TV and film, she may acquire new or replacement friends more readily than I, but I assure you it's probable or possible to make new friends over sixty. Whoop and I met after I was sixty.

How did we meet, you ask? Although neither of us is a fashionista, we met at the Ralph Rucci Fall 2010 collection show during New York Fashion Week, a time when international fashion collections are shown to buyers, the press, and the general public. Ralph is an American couture fashion designer, an artist, and my friend of many years. While it's very exciting to see all the new designs at New York Fashion Week, it's a *máximo* stressful event for designers!

I remember every detail of the evening, starting with the flash of cameras from the roster of fashion photographers trying to catch Whoopi, Martha Stewart, Fran Lebowitz, André Leon Talley (American editor-at-large of *Vogue* at the time), and many long-standing big-name clients all wearing Ralph Rucci to compliment his talent. Ralph has always attracted customers of a "certain age," partly because the clothes he designs, with their sculptural look and intricate handwork (sheer paneling and his innovative use of fabrics), are, like art, quite a healthy investment.

Okay, back to me and Whoop. Seating arrangements at these showings are plotted and re-plotted over weeks to get journalists and major customers placed just so. The seating, meetings, and greetings of the cognoscenti at these runway showings are a large part of the events, and Whoop, being a celebrity, was of course seated in the front row. I was scarcely visible, buried in the second row across the way.

Ralph really knows how to present a line of stunning, hollow-cheeked, leggy models in dazzling clothing. Everyone erupted into cheers and clapped wildly at the end of this gorgeous show—one of Ralph's best!

But before the showing began, my cousin Countess Lucienne von Doz spotted Whoop in the front row and brought her over after learning that Whoop's seating location was also due, in part, to a minor orthopedic problem. I had retired as an orthopedist by this point but was able to recommend some suggestions to alleviate her condition.

As happens with congruent beings, Whoop and I knew immediately that we wanted to spend more time in each other's company. We started by getting together at Whoop's annual blowouts on the

Fourth of July and Christmas, then gradually started to see each other on less formal occasions.

The more we grew into our "Broadship," the more we shared. Over the years we spent many dinners and holidays at her terrific home. These were happy times and helpful times of friendship—a new, over-age-fifty-five friendship.

If, as you get more and more into your Broad years, you think, *Phooey! I don't need new friends or their experiences*, that's your choice. But if you read something and think, *You know, I'd really like to try that*, then look into doing something new, and you'll eventually link up with new people too.

Remember that thoughts or statements you find interesting are often what initiate a new friendship. There are friends to be found when you come out of the shadows of your own mind.

It's been my experience that younger women might be afraid of becoming Broad, and that's why those in their forties and fifties don't approach us. The bias is noticeable. In these cases it's up to us Broads to show that the numbers don't signify (remember that chapter?).

My great bud Diane and I met when she was in her forties and I was in my eighties. She used to drive me into the city to buy apples at the farmers market, and we always got into conversations with people there. You never know; wherever you wander, you can make a friend if you have a common interest—even heritage apples. Consider this: the new is always refreshing. I introduced Diane to the cheese lady, the egg man, and my friend the beekeeper.

Social standards broaden with age, I find. I might not have considered the egg-and-butter man as a possible colleague in my younger years (not our kind, dear), but as you get older, you'll realize that the people around you are very much a part of your crowd. You're missing out if you don't broaden your horizons. A

Broad has to get off her bottom and make the effort with up-and-coming Broads. It's worth it—both for she who gives and she who receives. Broads have to educate their juniors. Open your mouth. Don't sit in the corner. Once an intergenerational friendship blossoms, it can spread from person to person.

Friendship
Through the Ages

DR. H

With the exigencies of WWII, when my immediate family was disassembled into several locales, I was unceremoniously relocated from Baltimore to the Shipley School in Pennsylvania.

Although I was thirteen at that time, I'd never been to Philadelphia, and I knew nothing of the all-girls venue in Bryn Mawr on the main line. More critically, I didn't comprehend that catching up educationally and socially would be a huge challenge for me. Many, if not most, of the students were from socially renowned families, while as a Jewish girl, I was a newcomer to their WASPy world.

We rose each day and donned the school uniform of short green wool tunics and starched white shirts over black wool long stockings, then we went through our predefined daily scholarly schedules. In this uniformed existence it was easy for friendships to flourish. I hasten to add that some un-friendships flourished as well, but the strict routine leveled out many intolerances and differences to livable proportions. Despite my educational and social deficits, I blended in after a couple of months without a problem. Perhaps it's universal that when one doesn't perceive difficulties, overcoming them is easier.

The next predetermined step after Shipley was a socially prominent college, followed by an equally prominent marriage. This was when, with the immediate uniformity of day-to-day schedules removed, my friendships began to dissolve, almost without exception.

I had a very good friend in one of my Shipley classes, a best-pal confidante type with whom I shared virtually everything. When we graduated, I went on to college, but my friend got engaged to be married. I was invited to the engagement party and other wedding events, but I knew no one and was often not really introduced, much less included, in her new circle. After the nuptials, my old friend simply had no time for me. The unity we had known evanesced, and I learned to appreciate the utility of uniformity.

I wish finding new friends was as easy in later life as it is at the school playground, which is full of high-spirited kids with endless imaginations and open hearts. Instead, when you're older, finding new friends takes considerable time and effort.

But in another sense, easy come is easy go. And fortunately, throughout my many careers, I've made friends who have endured the passage of time and sometimes distance and physical difficulties. Since I worked in theater for a number of years before my medical career, many actors, whose names are familiar to all, became friends. Many of them remained my dinner and also golfing partners after leaving the theater.

When I was seventy-nine years old, I moved to Pennsylvania, to the beautiful countryside full of horses, hills, and valleys covered with wide-cast wildflowers. It was here that a neighbor a few acres away dropped off a welcome-to-the-community bottle of champagne and the earnest message that if I needed anything, I should call her. I invited her over to share the bottle, and we've been friends for dozens of years hence. This chance meeting initiated my life's most cherished friendship with Diane Smith.

As a writer I tend to be fluent and detailed but lack organization. Fortunately, just down the street lived Diane, one of the most brilliantly organized people I've ever known. She became the organizer of every book I've written, with the exception of the novel I wrote while living in Paris before I met her. She's all anyone could wish for in a collaborator.

The best way I have made friends in my sixties and beyond is through common interests. You might start by looking around you, at those in your community who may be doing things that interest you, and joining in! Friendships tend to become not only the spice of life but the I've-got-your-back of existence.

Friendship takes time and a degree of deliberation. The good news is, when you're over age fifty or sixty, you may well have the leisure to seek out new friends and the time to spend with them. Their lives and interests may interest and enrich you.

On an interpersonal level, for many there's a certain kind of animal sense that tells you when someone is a foe, indifferent acquaintance, minor friend, or lifetime major pal. And oddly, this sense is highly developed in seniority. Use it, by all means, in addition to the other tools that can lead to new friendships.

Dress Like a Broad

DR. H

Whoop and I have gotten to the point in our careers where we often appear on-screen from the waist up. (Blessed be those of you with the tact to arrange this!) While I'm mostly on Zoom meetings, Whoop is, of course, sitting at a table on *The View*. The producers of her show do like to make an exception to show the audience her footwear. Granted, Whoop does the occasional head-to-toe fashion spread or personal appearances or films in wig and outré gowns, but hey, it's part of her job.

You don't have to retire from fashionable, appealing, or even sexy apparel because you're over sixty. Beware: if you do, you'll be asking for a pitying look, slower service, and never a "Good to see you."

There was a time in my life when fashion meant a lot more to me than it does now. In my teens, during the early 1940s, my beloved grandmama subscribed to the Theater Guild's fall and spring seasons. They were renowned for presenting the cream-of-stage Broadway productions from the top playwrights and featured the most gifted performers. We traveled from Baltimore to NYC twice a year, attended matinee performances in suitable day dress, and then went back to our hotel where we bathed and changed into cocktail/informal dinner dresses before going out to one of New York's well-known restaurants for dinner.

When she could no longer travel, she encouraged me to follow the same tradition of presenting a New Yorker style to the world. So in the spring and fall I contacted Miss Bette, a personal women's dress shopper at Saks Fifth Avenue. I might have chosen Altman or Tailored Woman, but Saks had the reputation for outstanding women's retail fashions.

Miss Bette was from a breed of middle-aged women who'd spent years in fashion for these venues (*Women's Wear Daily* being the Bible). She was a fashion cognoscente, easily identifiable by her understated but highly styled clothes in subdued colors that never competed with those of her clientele. The Miss Bettes made sure that the latest issues of *Vogue, Elle,* and other magazines were on side tables within easy reach of their to-be-seated customers.

When I arrived for my appointment, Miss Bette took me to my own furnished, carpeted dressing room featuring several three-way full-body mirrors. She had picked out a rack of season-appropriate wear for daytime, cocktail, and dinner dress, as well as the coats to match. I remember pieces by designers such as Pauline Trigère, Geoffrey Beene, and Adele Simpson. Miss Bette always supplied me with the latest designer brands. I usually picked out about a half dozen dresses.

At that point coffee or tea was served, and after, the appropriate shoes were brought up from their departments. Then final outfit choices were made, the address of my hotel specified, a charge card rendered, and a yellow cab taxi called. To say that I was a young fashion plate would not be far from an accurate description. I was, in effect, ready for society, whether or not it was ready for me. And this persuasion or habit persisted through many of my middle years.

As the age of sixty has become the former forty-five (actuarially and medically), seventy and eighty are very much still in the game of what to wear and how to wear it, if our outfit choices are cleverly executed.

Our figures likely have changed, but they don't have to be hidden within oversized, sexless envelopes of clothing. One thing is certain: never let someone else approve what you wear. If you give yourself the chance, you are the best possible stylist for you. And if this hasn't always been the case, start making it so now!

Go out feeling you're giving the public something chic or fun or just plain colorful and different. Head turning is the desired effect.

When I worked in theater, most of my time was spent liaising between actors and the public, so I had to develop a "look" that projected authority but did not compete, necessarily, with what my stars wore. I wound up adopting a uniform. It consisted of a pair of black jeans, a black cashmere V-neck sweater, black sneaks (sneakers), and a triple strand of cultured pearls. Now, as an Old Broad, I give myself a little more leeway, but in essence I wear custom-made shirts over custom-made pants and still lots of jewelry. Plus headgear consisting of custom-inscribed baseball caps and berets in all the colors of the rainbow.

A final note: Broads, please do your best not to shuffle, even if it means getting support from a walking aid or another person. I once used a nineteenth-century sword that concealed my agate-topped cane as a walking aid, and I still have it somewhere about the house.

Arthritis is a killer when it comes to style, but lift up your head, look the world in the eye, and say internally, *Ready or not, here I come—someone to notice and admire!*

Julius Caesar, conqueror of the then known world, once said for his spectacular appearance on a scene, *"Veni, vidi, vici"* (I came, I saw, I conquered). Broads should affirm the same!

Dating (An Entirely Different Subject)

WHOOPI

∞

Okay, I don't know about you all, but I've found that dating is problematic. I mean, it sounds like a good idea, but let's really examine what it means, particularly in light of the COVID-19 pandemic.

Dating during COVID-19 means Zooming with people. It's tough enough Zooming with people you know, but now you have to figure out how to Zoom with people you don't know. So, the question is: Do you get dressed up to Zoom? Do you have to put on makeup? Do you have to put on lipstick? Do you have to wash your face? What do you have to do?

I'm talking to you, ladies. I mean, there are lots of questions that come up with this because you know if you had to put on heels and other stuff, you'd be bitching all the way to the door—so you can only semi-bitch when you are having a first date on Zoom. Because really? A little lipstick? They don't know what else is going on. You could be buck naked (well, I don't know if you could be *buck* naked, but you could be naked down low because no one would ever know). And it's great because they're there in their space. You can "tee-hee" all you want to, and it's fantastic. The problem comes when people want to meet.

Now, you can only use the pandemic as an excuse for so long because if you start a relationship, you have to meet the person. And then you have to figure out, *Am I going to get in bed with this person?* and it's exhausting. So then you think, *No, I just want to Zoom for the rest of my life.* I will marry someone on Zoom as long as I don't have to see them. I don't want them in the bed, and I don't want them rolling over. (It's hot; you get hot in the bed next to people. I know you're supposed to enjoy cuddling, and I know for people who are married, sharing a bed is a wonderful thing, but as a non-married person, I get to the place where I think, *Why are you in my bed? You need to go home to your house.*) And I don't want to have breakfast the next morning and have someone in my business and looking at my stuff. I'm not into it.

Now, that might just be because I am a singular soul. Some people are not meant to be in relationships; I think that may be my case, but for everyone else, if you're going to date, it really is a commitment, and you're going to have to make a decision. People want to be in pairs, and if you don't pair well, you gotta start out with that knowledge and be up front about it.

So, I tell my dates, "I will Zoom date you, but I'm not gonna sleep with you. Not because you're not cute, but because the idea of having to smell someone else in my bed—it can't play." That's just me, and I'm consistent.

Dating (Another Take)

DR. H

ating is a word that we generally associate with teenagers and on through those in their twenties, thirties, and forties. Actually, teenagers claim dating as a rite of passage from childhood into adulthood. And a certain loss of social status descends on an individual if they are romantically unsuccessful, no matter their age.

As the younger members of the family tend to view it, dating is not an over-sixty—much less over-seventy!—pursuit. By and large, if they consider the subject at all, children think of their parents or older relatives as having already had their turn and therefore being in a place to pursue other, more "age-appropriate" activities than dating.

Is that "where it's at" for us over sixty? I think, fortunately, this is not the case—nor should we be talked into this idea!

Fact of the week: just because the younger generation thinks so doesn't mean you're on the shelf.

Actually, dating for those over sixty is a relevant, exciting, and often challenging activity. Think about it. The desire for romantic attention and companionship doesn't disappear. On the contrary, aloneness may create a new emotional or social need if you've lost a marital companion through divorce, outliving, or any other reason.

But dating as an Old Broad is not driven by the same social standards or parental pressures young people face. For instance, whereas teenagers tend to seek those "alike," age often permits far wider and more interesting partner choices. Because we are more experienced and knowledgeable about people and ourselves, we generally know what we like, what we'd like to learn more about, and what we absolutely don't care for.

I think it's high time we seniors disabuse our juniors of the idea that dating is age inappropriate. Our age is not a problem. Rather, the problem we need to resolve is where and how to find suitable candidates for dating.

The idea of going on a date to the movies or a show, for example, is wonderful for those of us over sixty. Not only will the date itself give us pleasure and enjoyment, but it will also lead to the secondary pleasure gained from making the effort to dress up and generally spruce up our personalities.

Indeed, dating is likely to produce a welcome break from your daily routine. The fact that we may anticipate or look forward to a date is fun in and of itself.

But if we decide that we are going to date, we have to accustom our younger family members or even friends to the idea. They have to realize that it's okay for us to look for affection or attention outside our immediate circle. What if they don't agree? They don't want you dating after grandpa dies? Tell them it's your life. Period.

You may find that dating as an Old Broad is different from what you experienced as a young person, when dating often implied sleeping with your date. Now it's maybe yes, or something more resembling mutual like or companionship. You and your date are free to define the relationship any way you'd mutually like. But don't forget the entrancing prospect of a new lover, if that's your wont (or want)!

So, what do we look for in an over-sixty date?

- Personal compatibility or the companionship of someone with a different life experience (this could be a neighbor, friend of a friend, or someone you meet at church, temple, or another social group)
- A fun occasion (concert, party, event) to share
- The possibility of a continuing association
- A reason to buy something new, or at any rate dress up
- The opportunity for admiration, interest, or respect

Where and how do we find these dates?

Let me start with the not-so-great idea, as it is the obvious and instantly doable:

Dating services may seem like an easy way to go, but sites like eHarmony, Match, and SilverSingles, while free at first, can become costly very quickly. Also, you must be aware of the potential for false promises and too-perfect biographies. The virtual has its pluses but also its negatives. By the time you've paid your initiation and possible individual introduction fee, you may be matched with someone who is less than desirable or even acceptable and *often not a peer in the broadest sense.* Okay, enough said. Dating services can be problematic. Approach with caution. Watch out for the face and form divine but feet of mud.

What then? Above all, don't sit at a bar nursing a wilted martini hoping for a chance encounter. In addition to nearly often being a waste of time, doing so may produce a false impression or even evoke a less than desirable approach. Think about the image. And the possible hangover the next day.

But there are many more appealing ways to meet people:

- Your church or temple may have groups such as book clubs or other special interest gatherings that appeal to you and to people of like interests.
- Your neighborhood, especially in a gated community, may sponsor specific social/meeting events or dances where you may find a date.
- Your married friends may know friends, or, if open-minded, your family members may know a peer (a decided advantage).
- One of your other friends may have a suitable acquaintance. All of these personal introductions imply a certain screening process, however informal, that may be positive in finding your fit.
- If you already belong to a group, like, say, aquatics or golfing, try going out with the group to restaurants you haven't tried before (especially during restaurant week) and getting to know the people in the group better.
- If you have a dog, try meeting people at the dog park. You'll already have an important area in common, and chances are that someone who loves their dog knows how to give and share love with another sentient being. (Apologies to all you turtle, fish, llama, and cat lovers who also may qualify!)
- And here's one more thought: you may have to look no further than the chair opposite yours. Suggest that you both get dressed up and go out on a date. You may be surprised and really pleased with the result and the easy settlement of an exact date for the date.

So, what do I have to say about the idea and opportunities of dating after sixty, seventy, or eighty?

It strikes me as a very good idea indeed!

It also occurs to me that the coming state of creation of humanoid robots, with perfect human appearances, speech, skin, and body texture (immediately responsive beings), is mind boggling.

A robot's conversation is initiated and controlled by you. It can literally be turned on or off at your will. Apologies to my coauthor who has a different view of dating, but I think there's something to consider here, and I await someone in a younger generation to write a full piece on robot romance.

Sex Over Sixty?

DR. H

You bet! Probably not the same sex you practiced at twenty or even fifty. And likely there will be needed (or wanted) modifications. But cardiologists say sex is one of the most valuable (not to mention enjoyable) exercises for their postcoronary patients. The only precondition to having sex after a heart attack is that you must be able to climb a set of at least fifteen stairs without getting dizzy, breathless, or experiencing chest pain of any sort. Not too demanding. I did six steps today, I'll do seven tomorrow, and when I get to the full flight? Look out below!

A well-versed poet observed that variety is the spice of life. And that aphorism is perfect on two counts to suggest the nature of sex over the age of sixty: it acknowledges both the length and history of your prior sex life and hints at many possible variations to come!

One caveat (not actually as strong as a warning) for those who have a significant degree of arthritis of the lumbar spine: missionary position, probably one of the most frequently employed for sex by the younger set, may be a problem. I don't think I have to elaborate on this if you are one of the many over sixty who have a wanky back. But for clarity, extension of the spine usually evokes a degree of pain. Instead, you might want to see what can be done side by side or even with someone sitting.

So, are there any pluses to sex over sixty? I think so.

First, there are no worries about unplanned pregnancies. Therefore, there's no need for condoms or other forms of birth control that may interfere with spontaneity and thought-free enjoyment. However, be sure to have a conversation about any positive (or for that matter, negative) experiences with STDs.

Second, the familiarity with your partner allows you to express aloud if something is uncomfortable or ineffective. For a newbie, it is not only acceptable but desirable to set ground rules appropriate to each participant prior to the activity. These may be some of the most interesting conversations you as a participant will ever experience.

Third, more inventiveness may be called for. A visit to a neighborhood sex shop, for instance, may be a fun shared event. Among the effective and fun toys, check out some of the aides or devices. Voice-activated dildos, positional pillows, and pre-sex lubricants are among the most popular items.

Fourth, when you were part of a younger couple with many daytime responsibilities, sex may have been limited to the nighttime. Even sex of the "wham, bam, thank you ma'am" variety. For the older practitioner, daytime makes more sense, as the body may be fresher and the house warmer. And your own kids are out working or doing their own thing, so privacy is easy. If you're a sexual yelper, no one will come rushing in fearing they need to call 911— or the police! And there is more leisure time to enjoy each moment for both parties as there are fewer time constraints. I'm not alone in appreciating this benefit. The French have a name for a romantic afternoon encounter (often accompanied by a glass or three of wine): *"l'heure bleu."* A well-known perfumer, Guerlain, created a very seductive scent by this name.

Traditional visual and auditory stimulants at any age to sex are the multitude of porno films and toys, many featured on virtual sex sites. If you haven't explored what effect they may have, there's no reason not to give it a try, particularly with a willing partner. They may evoke interest in any partnership, either temporary or more permanent. I refer to teledildonics as a technical sex tool and the game *Wheel of Foreplay*. Both are part of the digital world. Personally speaking, the game is fun, but I think the technical program may interfere with warmth, individual intimacy, and the easy adjustments of old-fashioned sex. And isn't this what we often look for in satisfactory sex? But I am, after all, old-fashioned in some ways. However, be careful because there's a lot of troubled or troublesome material being promulgated via the virtual. If something strikes you as really odd or even weird, my suggestion is don't engage!

For most of us, sex over sixty is not an everyday happening. Regardless of when and where you may choose to engage with your partner, here are some tips that will may make this a more pleasurable experience, starting with foreplay. Always remember that mutual masturbation is a form of foreplay. This can play an enjoyable part, especially if one or both partners have size or agility problems.

Maybe, for a special occasion, try dressing up, down, or many which ways instead of simply stripping off whatever you put on in the morning. (Apologies to those of you whose forte is inventive sex.)

Lastly, while visiting a sex shop or adult shop, ask for a copy of the *Kama Sutra* (translated, of course), preferably in paperback if you plan to use it as a reference during a session. You might try at least a few of the suggestions that appeal and are not overly pretzeled.

Sex in your seventies or eighties will most likely be a matter of performance versus expectation, and it is undoubtedly not the sex of your thirties, forties, or even fifties. Remember: all is grist that's brought to the mill.

You may encounter sniggers from your juniors, friends, and, yes, family as well as foes at the mention of your sex life. As for those who snigger, one day, they, too, may meet their moment of no-go-sex or some other earthy activity. Then one can only sympathize with their tears of regret!

There will come a time when physical disabilities defeat the desire for sex. Be prepared, and accept all you're able to until the day this happens. Enjoy all that you've had. Always remember to thank your partner.

And until then, a little poke can turn the summer day warm *and sunny*! And—last word—as Mae West quipped, "If you don't have a good partner, you'd better have a good hand."

Sex over sixty? You bet!

Is There Life After Jimmy Choo?

DR. H

At some point in your shoe-wearing career, you may have worn a pair of Jimmy Choo (or Manolo Blahnik) "creations," as I've heard them called. If you haven't worn them, at least you know what they stand for in women's shoes—the most stratospheric heels, for equally stratospheric prices, in eye-popping colors, finished off by the shortest vamps created by shoemakers anywhere and at any time.

Inherent to the proposition of wearing one of these creations is a sizable risk factor of slipping and falling. Most Broads who wish for style in their footwear are smart enough to give the above features at least a second thought before employing.

Among my favorite patients were those who came in with foot problems clearly needing surgical help (most commonly due to bunions and hammertoes). My own criterion for corrective surgery was significant, even if the patient had pain walking short distances. Actually, as a responsible surgeon, I always wanted a solid reason to do surgery. Cosmesis alone didn't cut it for me.

My first suggestion to my patients with foot problems was to change their footwear to a lower heel and a more accommodating last. They were to totally do away with bragging rights over their heel size. If there's ever been a cogent saying anent the shoe, it's: "Pride goeth before a fall." Literally, the wrong footwear can be more than partially causative in a trip or tumble.

One of the most common causes for surgery is bunions. A bunion is an imbalance of the forefoot, which develops as the foot matures—regardless of footwear. Fashionable, tight shoes encourage but do not cause them. Hammertoes are more causally related to the fashionable shoe.

By the way, with regard to surgery in women over sixty, doctors employ different techniques than those used for younger patients. I thought the simplest pain-relieving surgery was the way to avoid possible complications for this group. Whether you choose to go with an orthopedic surgeon or a chiropodist (podiatrist), it is fair to describe bunion surgery as major surgery in a "minor anatomic area."

As an orthopedist, I will grant that a podiatrist (chiropodists) who has graduated from an accredited podiatric residency may be the best way to go. You may want to go with a podiatrist who does hospital-based foot surgery. If you choose an orthopedic surgeon, be sure to inquire how many procedures he or she does per annum. While repetition is never a guarantee of proficiency, you may want to go with the surgeon who does many rather than few.

In my practice I did many major joint replacements, being well trained to do them. Secretly, I loved foot surgery and welcomed the problems of the under-prized foot. The expectations of the joint replacement patient are well known and well celebrated, but I often found that the patient who'd had a successful bunion or hammertoe correction was the one who brought flowers to my secretary and various goodies to me as well as quantities of recommendations!

SENIOR SHOE CONSIDERATIONS

First, keep your heels well under three inches, unless you plan to sit in one prominent chair for the evening and change in the ladies' room before you have to cross the floor to visit the food table, dance, or hail transportation home.

Second, don't wear the same shoes all day. Believe it or not, sweaty feet are an invitation to medical problems including fungal infections. Prolonged use of a single pair of shoes is asking for trouble, so change your shoes at least once daily. While you're changing them, take a good look at the anatomy and color of your foot as well as any growing sore spots and painful calluses. Don't forget to check in between your toes. You might also want to consider getting a foot massage, a positive pleasure if there ever was one, at your next pedicure.

Walking barefoot is actually quite good for your foot health. In the summer, going barefoot on a safe surface is fine, and I think you will recognize the features of any locales that aren't safe for this kind of walking. As a plus, think of the exercise your toes get when you walk barefoot, especially in sand.

Be aware that as the seasons change, your footwear should modify to accommodate the weather conditions, especially rain and snow. I particularly favor woolen socks under foul-weather gear; rayon or other blends may cause your feet to sweat without the ability to breathe or absorb the moisture.

There are plenty of choices for attractive shoes and lots of positive things to do for your feet. The makers of what used to be the exclusive realm of sports footwear have become a terrific source of color and style (and also often price). Their offers go far beyond "tennies."

In time you'll need to move beyond Jimmy Choo, Louboutin, and other fashionista foot mavens to something like care and sanity in women's shoes. If you care for your feet, they will reward you with loyal silence, service, and safety.

Girdles

DR. H

Remember that great scene in *Gone with the Wind* when Mammy (Hattie McDaniel) is using all her considerable strength to tighten the laces of a girdle on Vivien Leigh as Scarlett O'Hara? While Scarlett clings to a bedpost for stability, Mammy says between loud gasps, "You done had a baby, Miss Scarlett and you ain't never going to be no 18.5 inches again. Never. And there ain't nothing to do about it." The scene closes before the girdle ever does.

I've had ninety-two years to observe female fashion, and the foundational garments that push, lift, and mash a woman's body into desirable shapes. My grandmama was born in the late 1800s, and my mother was born in 1905. Both wore a girdle all their lives, not for complete figure control but perhaps for some minor figure enhancement and as a basis for securing their stockings.

When I turned fourteen, Mother took me to one of the eminent Baltimore ladies' undergarment shops. It was almost as a rite of passage for girls of my social class. To put this into perspective, the legal age of marriage in Maryland at the time was sixteen.

Mother and I had discussed the upcoming first girdle on several occasions, and each time I had expressed growing, if polite, opposition to it. So, despite my love for and usual desire to please my mother, on that dreadful day when she took me to the most upscale shop in the city, I finally said, "Mama, you will have to fetch all the shop girls to get me across this or any other undergarment store door."

The refusal was the first of my life and, as the beginning of typical teenage rebellion, led to others. I did accept that compromise we all acceded to for a while: garter belts. But it was always just one more undergarment to put on and adjust.

The demise of the girdle and the advent of pantyhose arrived simultaneously, perhaps aided by the demands of WWII for rubber (an innate element of girdles). For those of you who remember, rubber was severely rationed as the military had first dibs. When the war ended, the demand for girdles disappeared, never to be returned, and was universally replaced by pantyhose.

More recently, spandex garments have entered the fray, based on an ergonomic concept intended for athletes. And yes, these clothes come in large double-digit sizes, but not infrequently with an unintended sausage roll at the waist, back, or thighs.

There descend upon you times—weddings, anniversaries (especially yours), special appointments, showers, you name it—when you're an important feature. A must appearance. "A spotlight shines on our . . ." These are the times when you go to your closet looking for something special, or at least suitable, to wear, only to discover when you put it on that it lacks an inch and a half inch of closure. You have few choices in these situations. First, refuse the invitation with a made-up conflict of interest? State you're going to be out of town for three months? Or consider admitting the onset of a chronic bodily elimination condition? (Heaven forfend!)

Second, you may also contemplate whether there would be any way to keep your back to the wall or sit in a high-back chair throughout the occasion. But you know that sooner or later, you're going to have to rise, either to speak, twirl on the floor, or, minimally, acknowledge someone. So, what are we Broads to do without the use of girdles? If you're bound by time constraints, take some advice from Charles James, the renowned fashion designer of the midcentury whose work inspired Gianni Versace, Christian LaCroix, and Zac Posen in the present era. To clients faced with this dilemma, he said, "Wear it with style as if it's the latest." (Yes, this sounds like the story of the emperor's clothes, but attitude goes a long way on a given occasion.)

You know that kids can go on an absolutely "no food for days" routine to drop quantities of pounds (accepting that the weight will come back on immediately when they start to eat again). But this approach is a health no-no for you as a more senior citizen.

All kidding aside, you either refuse the invitation, mash yourself into spandex, or go shopping.

SWIMSUITS

A brief history of bathing suits (all dates circa):

- Prehistory: Nude
- Roman Empire: Public baths, togas/tunics (men only!)
- Nineteenth century: All-covering costumes, matching hats, and stockings
- 1900 to 1940: Woolen bathing suits, bathing caps
- 1940 to 1950: Two-piece garments for women, with or without a cap
- 1960 to 2000: Ever-shrinking bikinis

- 2000 to present: Privates-covering mini square of fabric, with or without a ribbon-sized breast cover (essentially, we're back to nude)

"By the sea, by the sea, by the beautiful sea."

Excursions

DR. H

I love to wander—always have. I'm curious, usually wondering what's behind the curtain, around a corner, or where a road may lead. I've always felt that when the body wanders, so, too, does the mind. And that's not a bad thing; it's like finding purpose in having no purpose at all. What a treat to find interesting things in places you would never expect to. Doing so seems to make the places special.

There were many times during my years of medical practice when no one could find me over my lunch hour. Then when I returned, I'd share about a fascinating thing, person, or bookstore I found on the streets of New York City. These excursions allowed me to experience new things and opened the door to happenchance, which, at the end of the day, made the day notable.

What are the differences between SoHo and NoHo? Not many NYC residents can tell you, but after many excursions, I can. When you wander, the differences emerge. Both neighborhoods are partially residential, with areas converted from old factories or warehouses. But NoHo features restaurants and food merchants; SoHo features clothing. I visited many shops and restaurants north and south of Houston Street (the "Ho" part of the names in the areas). These voyages into the unexpected created many experiences and subsequently filled me with knowledge and memories.

So, in essence, what I'm driving at is no excursions equal limitations, FOMO (fear of missing out), or other negatives. Excursions allowed me to experience new things and kept the days more interesting!

We can all remember the excitement of piling into field trip buses as kids, anticipating a day away from school with a fun visit to a science museum, the zoo, or a historical site. Parents and teachers endured the interruption to our daily routines because they felt these experiences played an important role in the mission of creating well-rounded citizens.

So, from one well-rounded citizen to another, aging well is really all about connections, continuous learning, and being socially active at all ages! Excursions, events, social outings (if following COVID-19 safety protocols), or even just video or telephone calls can help us stay social and part of the community. They also help stimulate the brain, improve sleep, and are a lot of damn fun and good for us!

Now, I grant you, excursions as such may be limited by various Old Broad conditions or ailments. But there's a secondary way to have it all. Describe a mission and then send your grandkids off— with money, if needed—to accomplish the excursion. Never question the value of what you're doing for them.

I have a nephew who I took to several operas, a number of Broadway plays, and any number of top restaurants (and yes, the relationship was in the general category of Auntie Mame) when he was still at a very tender age. I got to spoil him; his parents had the hard labor of the rest of his learning.

When we visit now, he may well say something like, "You know, Aunt M'Ellen, I did something yesterday that reminded me of when you took me to . . ." When he brings up these memories, I can almost hear the tunes or voices and see the actors. If such recollecting doesn't make your day, fellow seniors, what could?

Finally, as to personal excursions, I can say with a certain up-manship in the neighborhood, "I was there and heard Pavarotti sing *Rigoletto*," or "Remember when we were at the opening of *Hair*?"

GOING ABROAD AS AN OLD BROAD

When we think of excursions, what we want to avoid is isolation and loneliness at *all* costs. Here is a little advice I can offer:

Have a Routine
I start my day with reading. I love the *Economist*, although some-times, I have to read and reread so I get the full context of the articles. Then I walk around, stretch, and have my breakfast. I am fortunate that I am still working (as an author), so virtual Zoom meetings and writing things like this book take up a great part of my day. But I also make sure I have time to get out (with a driver) for errands and social lunches—again, ensuring my activities are safe in light of COVID-19. This routine helps me feel connected and keeps me contributing.

Reach Out
I didn't know about Zoom until COVID-19 hit, and boy oh boy, how wonderful is this tool! I learned how to use it and today use it several times a week for meetings with my editors and friends. Now, if you don't Zoom, no biggie; just use your phone to speak

with friends, or maybe try FaceTime to connect with friends and family or even people with whom you have lost touch. This is the perfect time to reconnect. And guess what? They may just love hearing from you and may need a nice pick-me-up!

Okay, now my favorite tip . . .

Try Something New

This can be anything from learning an instrument to bird watching! Then there's photography, knitting, fishing, going to museums, and more. There are so many online tours as well. You can virtually visit places like the Louvre, the Metropolitan Museum of Art, or even the Grand Canyon (as long as you're not afraid of heights!).

Look, the world is a fascinating place just waiting for you and your next excursion, whether it be by plane, car, bus, or online. The most important thing is to plan for one and never be bored! Remember, the journey of a thousand miles begins with one step.

PART THREE
Broad Bones

An informed patient is part of the solution,
not part of the problem.
DR. M. E. HECHT

THE ACHES AND PAINS HOUR

PATIENTS AS JUNIOR PARTNERS

FOUR EARS PLUS ONE NOTEPAD EQUALS A WINNER!

A VISIT TO THE DOCTOR: NEVER A ONE-WAY STREET

FEAR OF SURGERY FROM A SURGEON'S POINT OF VIEW

MEDICAL SECOND OPINIONS

GETTING CHOOSY

FEAR OF ANESTHESIA

DON'T GET RIPPED

YOU AND YOUR EARS

DENTAL PHOBIA

The Aches
and Pains Hour

WHOOPI

∞

had no idea how many annoying little things would start to happen to my body as I aged. Not like things where you think, *Oh,
haha, that's so cute!* No. I'm talking about things where you get
up and think, *Did I just leave my coccyx on the chair?* Because suddenly, you've got an ache. I can tell you, I've never ached so much
as I do these days.

I can tell you when it's going to rain, when it's going to snow, if
there's a fire watch in some state. I can tell you what trees are
blooming. I'm telling you, I am a font of physical information now.
When I stand, I sound like I am playing clackers; my knees make
so much noise, and I think, *Did I just break something? Is something
wrong here? Should I be sounding like this?* Apparently, yes, I should.

I guess all the air that you let off in your life, thinking you're
gonna be clear of it, gets into your joints, and when you stand up
or crack your knuckles, it sounds like dynamite. Exploding! Except
muffled, 'cause only you can hear it in your body. In any case, some
of this will make sense to you—not all of it, but I never said I was

going to make sense. I simply said I was going to let you know about aches and pains and things.

Arthritis. Arthritis! I have a touch of arthritis. Moving my neck around, moving my shoulders, I have bursitis. I mean, I have a lot of "itises." I think if my body didn't remind me all the time that it's changing, all this change would be a lot easier to take. But your body can't help it; it's like a bad friend that just has to let you know, "Oh, I see your teeth are loosening up in your mouth, and you can't chew the way that you could. And what's that clicking sound when you chew? You can't bite an apple?"

When you realize your body's not your best friend anymore, that you and your body used to be able to get away with all kinds of stuff but can't now, your body tells you everything. It has a big mouth, you have a bigmouth body, and there's nothing you can do about it because it's the only body you get. So you gotta take care of it, even though it's telling on you.

DR. H'S TWO CENTS

From where I sit at ninety-two, short and sweet will make you the most popular girl on the street! If you feel you really must (want to, wish to, need to) talk about your aches and pains, here is a behavioral plum. I guarantee it will make family, friends, and even the unsuspecting happy. This exercise can be called the "Aches and Pains Hour"—but you may only use it once a day, all-inclusive and done! Pick one hour and one person in the household or social group to be your listener. No further mentions, hints, or demos! Get it all out of your system. In one go.

I like to do my hour just after breakfast. My household has gotten trained. You may need to do an introductory session where you set a time that's good for all.

Patients as
Junior Partners

DR. H

Take it from an insider: medicine in the US of A has changed a lot in these past years. And not entirely for the better. Yes, coverage has improved, but it's questionable if the overall quality has done likewise.

One of the biggest changes I've observed is a process of diminished individual care. With that lack of individual attention, the medical-industrial machine relies on collecting and using digital information to help patients make medical decisions.

The problem with a patient relying on computer algorithms is that the patient, by and large, hasn't got a medical education. So how can they discern helpful from non-helpful or discern reliable, accurate, and unbiased from ad hominem sources? The lack of understanding causes nearly universal worry and fear, which practitioners detect in most patients.

In my view, there is an essential need for patient education as part of successful treatment. In my years as a health-care provider, I regularly saw a lack of understanding writ large on patients' faces, whether those patients were in the crowded venues of large city hospitals, being seen in top private medical clinics and practices, or, perhaps most overwhelmingly, waiting to go into an operating room. Not a pretty picture.

I can identify two primary factors that contribute to the patients' ill-equipped state ahead of any procedure: (1) patients' lack of basic education about the human body and (2) physicians' inability to communicate effectively with patients.

From first grade through college and even postgraduate study, we are taught many subjects (languages, literature, mathematics, and others), but no curricula contains courses or lectures on human anatomy or human physiology. Therefore, most people understand nothing of the manifestations of abnormalities (i.e., illness, malfunction, injury, or malignancy) in these areas. So when a physical malfunction occurs, reactions tend to range from intense worry to fear and even panic.

On top of this, physicians and surgeons, no matter how extraordinary their medicinal skills and knowledge of the human body, are not taught communication skills. And, I might add, they rarely have this skill in their general armamentarium!

It took me several years and several assignments to realize that patients' fearful reactions to treatment were not inevitable but, rather, might be remedied if the patients were treated as partners in their own care. I could convert a well-informed surgical patient into a junior partner and part of the solution in a proposed procedure. They simply needed to know what was amiss, what was to be done to correct it, and finally, what the post-surgical period was likely to include.

This practice of cultivating patients as junior partners was self-serving, too, as it had a demonstrably positive effect on my surgical success rate. Any surgery requires a team to make it successful. We know all about team members such as the surgeon, the

OR nurses, the gurney operators, and anesthesiologists, but we never talk about another critical member of the team: the patient participating in every part of the procedure. The junior partner.

How to become a junior partner:

1. When researching your condition online, use bona fide sources such as WebMD, National Institutes of Health, American Diabetes Association, Mayo Clinic, Drugs.com, MedlinePlus, Cleveland Clinic, and Family Doctor.org.
2. After all your research, keep an open mind to what your doctor says about your specific case—yours may not be a textbook case.
3. Employ the Four Ears (two of yours, and two of a companion's), One Notepad method. If you're confused, ask for a simplified explanation.
4. If in the end you don't feel informed or aided in the matter, as draconian as this sounds, remember there are many good surgeons performing the same procedure to be found. You can always take the bull by the horns and go to another office.

WHAT IF THE DOCTOR DOESN'T WANT A JUNIOR PARTNER?

You may not be able to find an in-network doctor with the right frame of mind to truly partner with you. You can still make the best of your situation by ensuring you understand what is going on to the best of your ability. To get a clear explanation from your appointed surgeon, ask for a description of the procedure and expected outcome in layman's terms, using words of one or two syllables.

Now here comes controversy and a caution: There's a lot of information and advocacy to be found online and even in physicians' booklets. Most patients may not have the information or education to separate the gold from the dross. Or even to avoid being taken in by fool's gold. So when, or if, you encounter this kind of marketing, check back with your MD or hospital for the genuine information you need. I particularly worry about digital and television ads for medications and procedures. Many I've seen proclaim things like, "Look, Ma, no hands in nature," and are misleading. Always check with a legitimate source—even when an advertisement's promise is really appealing.

Four Ears Plus One Notepad Equals a Winner!

DR. H

When I opened the Hecht Group for second surgical opinions in 1982, I established a new patient intake process that required patients to bring a friend or relative with them who could listen as coolly as possible to everything that transpired. I asked this friend/relative to bring a notepad, phone, or iPad to document everything they heard. We called this the Four Ears, One Notepad method of doctors' visits.

If the patient questioned the need for the extra ears and record keeping, my talented and assertive office administrator, Gloria, said, "You've dialed the office of a female orthopedic surgeon, and this is the way we practice. We think you'll find it suits."

Looking back on those years, I don't recall a patient who later said, "I felt my first appointment was off-putting."

We also asked patients to bring to their first visit a written medical history, as complete as they could make it, together with a list of medications they took on a regular basis. And although it took more effort on their part, we found that the presence of these records helped both doctor and patient avoid overlooking anything that might affect the treatment plan.

Even though the practice of medicine and of surgery has altered dramatically since then, I still wish all patients would follow my advice and bring another set of ears and a notepad to *all* doctors' visits. Think of it this way: if the standard patient visit is fifteen minutes, a patient stands to gain another fifteen minutes of listening, for a total of thirty, when a second set of ears is there to help.

The point of the Four Ears, One Notepad system is to enable yourself to *consider at leisure* the possibilities and process of the medical advice being offered. It really doesn't matter how small or extensive the proposed surgery or treatment plan is.

A Visit to the Doctor:
Never a One-Way Street

WHOOPI

OO

Some of my musings are shorter than others. Like this, for instance: a visit to the doctor must not be a one-way street. That's right! Because the doctor can tell you everything they need to tell you, but if you don't tell them what they need to know, they can't really help you.

So stop trying to be cute and courageous. It's time to tell the damn doctor what he or she needs to know. Okay? You're too old to be futzing around holding things back. Tell them what they need to know—it will make your life easier.

DR. H'S TWO CENTS

For anyone over sixty, a visit to the doctor can and should be optimized to both prevent possible upcoming trouble and treat current conditions. It's best to schedule doctors' visits as three-or-four-times-a-year events (not unlike the regularity of the seasons in spring, summer, fall, and winter). These visits can be either in person or virtual utilizing telemedicine, if lab work or physical examination is not critical.

I use the word *events* deliberately because a visit to the doctor should not be viewed as a chore to be ignored, avoided, or dreaded. And as an event, there are ways to take advantage of the visit by maximizing the benefits and extracting essential information about your health conditions and how to manage them, especially if a new medication has become available as a treatment or preventive. As a planned occurrence, the visit can also be a major tool of independence and control. And who among us doesn't relish these things at any age.

You make the difference. How you prepare and manage the visit is key. Organize your visit with the intention of getting the most out of it. Believe it or not, this will even help to organize your doctor! Remember, the doctor-patient relationship is a two-way street. You are in the doctor's office to report and learn about your health, and the doctor is there for the same reasons.

If you are prepared to participate and report your current state of being in an organized way, you'll gain the attention and interest of your physician. Especially if you come ready to describe and quantify what's going on. And, of course, you'll come with notes too (not relying on memory)! Consider reporting on the following:

- Have there been any changes in your recurrent conditions? If yes, when, how, and how severe were these changes? And did you do anything to modify and/or ameliorate your symptoms? If so, did your efforts work or not?
- Have you experienced any changes in your response to the medications your doctor has prescribed? Which medications are you are currently taking?

- Have you experienced any new signs or symptoms of illness or injury?
- Have you made any changes to your level of activity? If yes, what were the results?

INFORMATION, PLEASE

Your report to your doctor must not be a haphazard story. You'll prepare by writing a list, as short and to the point as possible, of each condition you want to review. Leave room for answers and suggestions. Then approach the doctor's response bearing in mind the following tips:

- Make sure you understand the answers and solutions your doctor provides, including the effects desired and any major side effects to be anticipated or reported. If your physician lapses into medicalese (doctor-to-doctor language), interrupt politely and ask for a patient translation. A simple, "Could you please repeat or reexplain that?" if you don't understand something does not constitute an imposition.
- Always bear in mind that it takes two to tango (as the saying goes). The white coat on one pair of shoulders doesn't automatically disable or devalue the importance of your full presence, understanding, and opinion.
- Write down the doctor's suggestions and keep your notes for future reference.
- If the doctor suggests something that is not possible or even probable for you to do, speak up so you both can come up with a modification or substitute.

- If you're going to engage in some kind of trial and report, be sure you understand the terms and establish when it's best to talk to the doctor. Many doctors tell patients that it's best to call at the end of office hours unless there's an emergency. As with your doctors' visits, write down the essentials before you call.
- Be sure to ask if there is any literature you can study at home—whether the doctor has a pamphlet or can refer you to a website.
- When next you come to the doctor's office, refer to your notes from the previous visit, noting whether suggested solutions have been helpful, so-so, or ineffective.

BEDSIDE MANNERS

Having good bedside manners is not a requirement for the doctor alone. It's something patients sometimes forget about or think of as not important, but it is! You want a doctor who approaches you with an easy manner, care, and forthcomingness. Likewise, your attitude and the way or manner of how you ask questions will help to elicit these traits. Your tone of voice can elicit great responses or terseness.

Above all, do not be defensive or demanding. The doctor is on your side. It is not always easy to be calm in the face of pain or disability. But your preparation to state the problem succinctly, and the calmness of your delivery, will solicit the best response from your physician.

WHOOPI'S TWO CENTS

When I was young, I didn't have the time or need to regularly visit a doctor. So all of this advice would have had no relevance. Now, as a beginning senior with TV and film commitments, it has become a must.

If you find some of these suggestions practically helpful, so will your physician, seeing that you have gone to the trouble of creating a real two-way street. I try to remember that I may be a star in a show or TV special, but my physician is a star in the doctor's office. The secretary and nurses are careful to observe this ranking, and so should you be, if you're smart.

But it's up to you to understand all that the visit evokes. If you do a good job of this, in the end, both the treater and the treated will be winners.

Fear of Surgery from a Surgeon's Point of View

DR. H

A re you secretly or not so secretly one of the legions of people who are truly frightened of "going under the knife"? Will you avoid surgery at any cost because you fear not surviving? Or are you one of many who suspect that much of what may be surgically proposed lies somewhere between unnecessary, unneeded, and mercenary?

If you answered yes to any of these questions, you are what most doctors would define as "surgery phobic."

Having said that, as an orthopedic surgeon, I cannot condemn such fears out of hand. Whether a surgery is elective or emergency, a patient's fear is not to be dismissed. But I have always believed that a well-informed patient who becomes part of the solution—and therefore a valuable junior partner—will have an unmistakably positive impact on the resultant surgery and will therefore begin to discover the cure for surgery phobia.

Surgery in the late nineteenth and early twentieth centuries fostered the idea of the white-coated Master Surgeon, after whom wards were named and whose rounds and words were open only to the most senior medical personnel on staff. Their dicta were quoted to junior surgeons and published in medical journals. That all went south after WWII, with its new techniques and battlefield surgical needs. In orthopedics the Master Surgeon just about vanished with the advent of Swiss (and other nations') advanced techniques.

In the 1960s and '70s, in part because of the coverage offered by Medicare, Medicaid, and so on, the medical world changed for the better in that outstanding talent was found and available on many levels. Doctors and surgeons had to come down from their pedestals and talk to human beings like fellow human beings almost by law, or at least Medicare law.

As a result, patients now have the ability to ask their surgeons intelligent, detective-type questions before entertaining the idea of an elective surgery (which most surgeries are). At a minimum, ask the what, how, and when of the procedure; what will happen if you do not undergo surgery; and what benefits and risks the surgery poses. If you have the answers to these questions, the prospect of surgery will get much more cut down to size, if you'll pardon the pun.

Beyond a doubt, information is the preferred and definitive answer to phobia. Remember as children how many of us feared walking into a dark room, no matter how familiar, because of an imagined threat or monster under the bed? But once you turned the light on, didn't that room simply become a room?

So to those of you who are surgery phobic, and for whom corrective or emanative surgery is warranted, I say help is at hand in the form of information, available and freely dispensed now by countless legitimate and appropriate agencies. The bedroom light can be turned on.

WHOOPI'S TWO CENTS

There are so many great ideas in this wonderful guide, but first you must make sure that if a doctor says you need to have surgery, you don't put it off. They're telling you for a reason.

Not everybody wants to spend your money. Not everybody is just trying to get over on you. But that's the world we live in; we think everybody's trying to fool us because no one seems to tell the truth and nothing seems to be what it is.

Yet when it comes to your health, you've got to make sure that you're taking care of business for yourself. There are people who really like you—and some who actually love you—depending on it.

UNNECESSARY, UNNEEDED, AND PERHAPS MERCENARY

No smart surgeon that I know indulges in unnecessary or iffy surgical procedures—if for no other reason than there are people, colleagues, and agencies who oversee surgeons' actions or to whom they may have to account for their practice. These include state medical licensing societies, confreres working in the same hospital, hospital surgical privilege committees, and physicians in medical insurance companies.

As to mercenary motivation, the era in which the Master Surgeon was paid huge fees has (by and large) passed because there are more and more surgeons capable of doing advanced procedures. It may also be noted that much of surgery today is paid for by third parties (medical insurance companies, either private or government sponsored, or medical health organizations). These organizations have more and more come to be the surgical payment monitors, setting given amounts of reimbursement for given surgeries and medical venues.

Medical
Second Opinions

WHOOPI

OO

Under normal circumstances, it's a good idea to get a second opinion. You need as many people as possible to tell you that you really need to get something done because you're hardheaded, and that comes with age. And maybe it's not just age; maybe you're scared 'cause there's a number attached to your name now, and you think it's closer to the back side of life than the front side (although people are living much longer than anticipated, so maybe we don't need to be as afraid). Regardless, you need to get to the doctor because if you don't go to the doctor and there is something wrong, it can kill you.

So I say, hear them all out. Hear as many opinions—from family, friends, and medical professionals—as you can and then figure out what to do. It's much better in the long run. Now, it's hard to get a second opinion about coronavirus. But in the words of Ethel Merman, "You either got it or you ain't."

A couple of years ago, I didn't feel good. I had a cough that seemed to last a year. And the day of You Know Who's second State of the Union address, I started thinking, *Boy, I really don't feel good, and this can't just be because I don't like him.* So, I called my trusty sidekick, who was in the city, and said, "Hey, I'm not feeling good."

He said, "Well, I don't know what to do except try to get to you, but it may take a while."

So then I called my other trusty sidekick, who said, "I'll be right over."

While I was waiting, we called another friend, who was in LA. After I described my symptoms, that friend said, "We're calling an ambulance." So, it was me at home, trusty sidekick number one, Tom, who was coming over from the city, trusty sidekick number two, Karen, who lived close by, and one of our favorite doctors on the planet, Dr. Jorge, in Los Angeles, calling an ambulance for me on the East Coast. You got it so far?

Okay. The first ambulance never made it. As a matter of a fact, I think they're still out there looking for the address. The second ambulance arrived. The emergency responder came in with his partner and a stretcher and said, "What's your name?"

I said, "Mary J. Ask me again and I'll tell ya the same." He chuckled, but I realized he was too young to understand the patter, so I told him my name.

He said, "Well, I'm going to take your temperature and vitals and we'll see what's happening." After he took my temperature he said, "Wow!"

So, I said, "Wow?"

And he said, "Wow." Then he took my blood pressure, and again he said, "Wow!"

And I said, "Wow?"

And he said, "Wow." Then he said, "I think we should probably take you to the hospital."

I said, "Well, I just really want to lay down, you know, and maybe I'll feel better in the morning."

He said, "I don't think that's a good idea." And that's when I knew I was much sicker than I'd thought. For the entire ride, he kept talking to me, and I realized he was trying to keep me awake.

My friend Karen drove behind the ambulance to the hospital. Tom was still on his way from the city. When I got to the hospital, the medical personnel took me into the emergency room, and they said, "Wow!"

I said, "Wow?"

And they said, "Wow." And then they took all kinds of tests before they came back and said, "We're keeping you. You have pneumonia in both of your lungs, and you're septic."

It was my turn to say, "Wow."

So, I spent a month in the hospital. I had my lungs drained and was woken up by more groups of people than when I was younger. (You know there are times when being woken up by a large group of people, even people wearing masks, is a great thing. Not when you're in the hospital.)

Double pneumonia and sepsis was a pretty clear-cut diagnosis. So, if you're not feeling well, don't fool around. Had I reached out to my friends or a doctor about that cough after two or three months, I might have saved myself the year and a half recovery.

DR. H'S TWO CENTS

Medicare and Medicaid no longer require a second opinion prior to elective surgery. But as a surgeon, I see getting a second opinion as an indispensable step for patients to take before having surgery. Whether you're having a bunion correction or a spinal disc removed, a nose job or a hip or knee replacement, you deserve a second opinion. Yes, doing so has become entirely a matter of your (the patient's) responsibility, but it's more than worth the effort to get one.

And don't worry about feeling awkward when you go to the appointment to get a second opinion. The new MD will know that you have booked the appointment as a second-opinion consultation and will applaud your smarts for doing so.

So, I hope I have sold you on the great value of a second opinion before you undergo elective surgery. And yes, "small symptoms" can develop into life-or-limb-threatening conditions.

It's really a matter of everyone listening to their bodies when they start to show unfamiliar or unusual symptoms. What is not normal is not normal and can *always* use an informed opinion.

Getting Choosy

DR. H

HOW A SURGEON MAY CHOOSE A PATIENT

Have you ever wondered when you enter a surgeon's office what the doctor may be thinking about you as a candidate for the procedure in which they specialize? Do you think they simply accept every patient who walks through the door? Think again.

When I started in practice, the females in my specialty were few and far between. Of those few, many were academics, which meant they were associated with teaching, not practicing. Patients expected, without exception, a male orthopedic surgeon to handle their cases. My office door and medical license read: M. E. Hecht, MD. Most patients did a double take as they were ushered into my office and learned that I was Mary Ellen Hecht. However, only a few refused to work with me.

When it came to elective cases, as an orthopedist who practiced for over thirty-five years I usually chose my patients. Or, to put it another way, within a few minutes of conversational exchange, I had a pretty good idea who would respond well to surgery, no matter how technically difficult the procedure. What was more, I could discern who would make a definite contribution to the successful outcome of the surgery. Emergency room referrals were, of course, a different situation where both the patient and I had no choice but to work together.

What did I and many of my colleagues look for in surgical candidates? Among the most important factors to me were to find patients who:

- were not fearful of asking about the odds of a positive outcome and the risks of a procedure
- asked how many joint replacements I did per year
- brought a complete account of their medical conditions and previous treatments
- asked how the surgery might impact their activities, especially sports
- asked whether they were an anesthetic risk
- asked how long they'd have to wait after surgery before returning to work or other usual activities

I think you get the idea—I always wanted a live wire as a patient, someone who wanted to be part of the solution. In short, I looked for active participants or, as I came to call them, junior partners (see the earlier chapter about this topic).

Joint replacement, unlike emergency surgery, is elective and involves choice—both the doctor's and the patient's. This means there were times when I put off patients who didn't meet my criteria, telling them: "My schedule is very full. Perhaps I can recommend another surgeon more available for you."

In general, I didn't accept patients who:

- said, in effect, "Just do it, Doc. I trust you." While this could be flattering, it's very worrisome and often leads to

noncompliance or unreasonable expectations after surgery
- feared "undergoing the knife" and had an overt aggressive or skeptical attitude
- found my name on a popular magazine's list of best surgeons
- obviously stopped listening when I talked of potential risks and their probability

HOW A PATIENT MAY ELECT A SURGEON

You should never consider yourself powerless in choosing your providers and in the ensuing discussions of treatment. The choice must be a two-way street.

There are obvious reasons to choose one provider over another. You may be more inclined to choose surgeons who are:

- recommended by your family doctor
- documented as specialists by the state medical society, etc.
- willing to educate you about the risks and benefits of the proposed surgery
- extensively trained in whatever procedure you're considering (check office walls for certificates and diplomas)
- able and willing to talk in your language (not in medicalese or important-sounding Latin diagnostic terms)

I think it's clear that the ideal surgical journey is a partnership between both the surgeon and the patient. And this is not only desirable but entirely achievable. So use choice wisely, and remember your surgeon may elect you as well as vice versa.

Fear of Anesthesia

DR. H

As to the very common fear of anesthesia, the science of anesthetic materials and techniques has become as developed as the advancements in open heart surgery, knee and hip replacements, and, yes, even facial surgery. Gone are the days of ether, with its possibility of violent allergic reactions on the table and postsurgical nausea and vomiting.

The procedures that require general anesthesia are pretty well limited to the abdominal, upper extremity, and cranial areas today. Moreover, the anesthetic agents currently used are quickly reversible, very effective in low doses, and often composed of a blend of opiates and sedatives—far safer than the general, heavy anesthetic techniques of the early nineteenth and twentieth centuries. Okay, fair is fair: the days of amputation under raw whiskey as the only available kindness are gone forever too.

As many procedures as possible are done under local or regional anesthesia in combination with sedatives—the perfect examples are hip or knee replacement surgeries that are done under a form of spinal anesthesia and a Valium-equivalent sedative.

These are calculated to be short acting, just enough to cover the length of the surgery.

If your doctor can perform a total knee or hip replacement with regional anesthesia and even talk to you for a bit during the surgery, doesn't that reassure you?

In other words, the risks and drawbacks of anesthesia from past centuries have been replaced with far more sophisticated—and much, much safer—techniques.

Armed with some of these observations, gathered through more than thirty years of medical practice, I hope you feel decreased anesthesia phobia.

No more ether, lessened post-op nausea and vomiting. The anesthesiologist today looks for you to have an anesthetic visit to la-la land and a gentle wake-up.

Don't Get Ripped

DR. H

Just a word about what goes with you as a patient immediately after you've had any type of surgical procedure. Virtually every patient is told to have rehab of some sort, but here are some things that you, as a suffering patient, must undertake to make a satisfactory recovery.

The most important instruction for you is to watch for possible trouble before you get involved with rehab. This includes looking out for infection and/or excessive post-op bleeding. Some less-obvious signs to be aware of include:

- increased swelling
- increased redness
- increased discharge or oozing from wound or surgical sites

Whenever you notice anything suspicious, take your temperature. Also do this automatically for the immediate day or two post-op.

If any trouble occurs, you're not ready yet for rehab. Contact your surgeon.

ANY POST-OP PAIN

Many surgeons go over this general information as a part of their treatment, but many surgeons are also not great communicators. So here are a few answers to common questions about post-op recovery.

1. *What do I do for some degree of inevitable pain?* Take mild analgesics, but if pain is persistent, call your surgeon.
2. *How much movement or activity should I try, and is there a progression path after surgery?* Don't be a hero; work to tolerance.
3. *Will starting rehab increase my pain?* Most likely, but the pain will lessen over time.
4. *How soon should the post-op pain begin to ebb?* This varies with each individual.

ON TO REHAB

Once you believe you've reached the point where rehab is a must, you may be tempted to follow an exercise program being promoted by someone with celebrity status. But beware!

Exercise programs, equipment, and instructors can be beneficial, simple, and straightforward. They can also be downright destructive, especially if ill-performed, too aggressive, or ill-advised.

It wouldn't hurt to ask your post-op exercise guru for credentials! The ancient Romans used the phrase *"mens sana in corpore sano."* It means "a healthy mind in a healthy body." Or, put another way, use your mind to spot trouble and insanity when talking about exercise/rehab choices.

Let's take a look at a variety of exercises you can do whether you're seeking to recover from a joint replacement or athletic injury or just looking for general conditioning. Almost any workout that promises you to "get ripped in thirty days" may indeed lead to rips, but not the kind you desire. When muscles and tendons rip, some might even need surgical repair!

I can't count the number of patients who came to me after trying out one of the latest featured workouts online. Many experienced strains or even increased pain and decreased range of motion in arthritic joints. When I asked them to show me the program that caused the problem or problems, I invariably saw instructors (fitness models) doing often extremely demanding exercises. With few exceptions, these instructors were very attractive, in full studio makeup, and dressed in the latest athletic fashions to display their admirable physiques. I need hardly tell you that almost all offered the program for a significant fee.

At this point the best I could do for my returning patients was to treat them conservatively by prescribing a period of rest and medication. Some required actual immobilization with braces or ACE bandaging.

As a patient considering rehab programs, seek first the worth and safety of what may be offered. Better still, check the program with your surgeon.

TYPES OF EXERCISE

You will want to incorporate several types of exercise into any rehab program, as each exercise is designed to help you achieve different ends.

Flexibility. Put all joints through a full range of motion plus flexion and extension. If you tend to be flexible, yoga is another possibility. But when you stretch, listen especially hard to your body; it will tell you (via pain) when a particular exercise or position is not for you. Yoga breathing and relaxation exercises are particularly good. Whichever method or exercise you choose to gain or maintain flexibility, the underlying principle of a slow execution (motion) is most beneficial.

Toning or Muscle Building. Work out with caution to fit your individual body and build, making sure your program is aligned to your body type and skill level. Be cautious when it comes to weight lifting, CrossFit, or any resistive work. The name of the game is to avoid strains, sprains, or, worse, permanent muscular damage. Above all, you over sixty must avoid being seduced into the serious error of believing in the "no pain, no gain" mantra. It simply ain't so. No way, no how!

Cardiorespiratory Work. Regular cardio workouts are important for older adults. This activity not only strengthens your heart and lungs but also gives you more energy and sharpens your mind. Among the best activities by far are swimming, ballroom dancing, and water aerobics. Cycling or fast walking are also good options. The worst and most harmful exercise is running, especially over long distances or on hard surfaces. It may boost your endorphins, but it also may induce serious knee strain, ankle wear, or injury over time, often requiring early joint replacement surgery.

FOR THE JOINT-CHALLENGED
OR ARTHRITIC

There's a bit of a problem for this group. Motion of the affected joint or joints generally produces pain. And that pain may last longer than the exercise. Or it may be evoked with minimal exercise. But if you choose to simply rest or sit all the time, you'll begin to experience pain with even less motion. So, exercise for the arthritic person is a problem but must be done regularly to whatever extent possible. What we call a paradox, no?

The wisest course of action is to consult a physical therapist for a series of designed exercises that allow for definite progress—even if that progress is slow. And then you need to exercise every day. I always suggested to my patients that it was okay to take a mild analgesic (such as TYLENOL or an equivalent) half an hour before an exercise session.

For the older or more incapacitated individual vis-a-vis the subject of exercise: physically, you may be limited and/or vulnerable to injury, but with years have come judgment or smarts. Use them to get the most out of the exercises you can do with impunity, understand why exercise is important to your being, and protect yourself from harm while you engage in activity.

Be sure to consult your MD to discuss what level of exertion and range of motion are safe for your body.

Here's a parting mantra to wrap up this discussion on exercise: do what you can today and try for a bit more tomorrow.

You and Your Ears

DR. H

Out of the hundreds of patients I saw in the orthopedic clinic at Kings County Hospital Center, I was struck by the expressions and tone of two specific patients. One was blind and had a charming way of talking and a peaceful expression. The other was hard of hearing. His face showed a constant anxiety and worry about understanding the information and proposed treatment he would be offered.

I found later that, almost universally, people who were blind emanated a seeming sort of acceptance and serenity, while those who were deaf or hard of hearing exhibited a real sense of despair and isolation. Perhaps the loss of hearing left them feeling more isolated and lonely.

The exact figures on hearing loss in the senior population have not been accurately computed. The diagnosis in this area is subjective. (Can you hear a little? Not much indoors? Only if someone speaks loudly? Not high-pitched voices? etc.) But if I suggested that well over 50 percent of people over sixty have some degree of hearing impairment, I don't think it would come as a surprise.

Hearing loss doesn't show up all at once; for most people, the onset is subtle. You may notice that speech from another room is not intelligible or words are hard to interpret when the person speaking is turned away from you. Or you may find yourself asking for frequent repetitions.

When I was small, my grandmama used to tease me about the acuity of my hearing. "You have the ears of a bat," she'd say. My bat-like hearing persisted until I turned eighty.

I knew that elderly loss of hearing was present in much of my maternal side (great-aunts and cousins in significant numbers), but nevertheless, when I recognized for sure what was going on, my immediate reaction was anger. I saw hearing failure as interfering with much of my life. I had, and, I suppose, still have, little tolerance for things that interfered with what I wanted to do. Many of you will relate to this.

I must admit that, for this egotist, there was just a drop of fear that the loss of hearing might become complete, and with it would come social isolation.

By the by, women seem to experience more of an emotional response to hearing loss than men. I'm not certain why, but there it is. Perhaps men don't find saying, "What's that you said?" or "Speak up!" as a personal problem but rather one to do entirely with the speaker.

FACE THE CHALLENGE

If you've got a grain of guts, you won't simply accept a growing hearing impairment. You will find it in you to inform and even discuss the problem with an intimate companion or member of the family or caregiver or—the person who can most help— your MD.

Then the next logical step will be to make an appointment with an ear, nose, and throat (ENT) specialist because the ear is part of an entire system, and you want to be sure your hearing alone needs amelioration. Next you will be referred for evaluation to an audiologist to determine the depth and character of your hearing loss.

None of the treatments available for hearing loss will restore your hearing completely. Rather, the question becomes how much can be augmented to restore a critical or functional level of hearing. There are two accepted ways of treatment. One is with a hearing device. The other, a cochlear implant surgery, is reserved for the very, very young. There may be other surgical solutions now under development, but a hearing device is the current best option for elderly loss of hearing. Ask an audiologist about rates of success and your choice of device.

I suggest you consider as a first step a hearing-enhanced telephone. There are many on the market. Even the Speaker function on your current instrument can help.

When it comes to defeating the feeling of isolation, you must take your vanity in hand and talk seriously to your family or caregiver. Ask them to address you face-to-face and increase the volume of their speech when speaking to you. If it's critical that you understand something, tell them they might even augment this with a written word or two. Don't forget your friends in the panoply of folks who must be informed.

Here's one benefit to hearing loss: much of what others talk about or what plays on the TV is inane, stupid, boring, or misinformative. You have a choice others may not have. Just shut your hearing device off and quietly win the attention battle.

Most importantly, remember that there's nothing in the least wrong with your brain or your ability to function except in this limited area. Reassure your family and friends of this by challenging them to a game of gin or hearts or solving the Sunday crossword puzzle or sudoku—and beat them silly!

Dental Phobia

DR. H

D ental phobia is almost a universal mental/psychological
pandemic! Now, if you're a hero, you've conquered it. I can
only imagine the smile that is on your face. If not, the
thought of visiting the dentist may send you into a scene of fear
and trembling. Even though mostly all dental procedures today
are achieved painlessly.

I wouldn't rate going to the dentist among life's pleasurable experiences. But it's not the horror show it once was. And, by and
large, you won't wonder, as you once might have, where and how
these pain merchants trained.

So, how did this phobia come to be? Let's look back at dentistry
derivation and history.

PHOBIA ORIGIN

Even as late as the early 1930s, when a few of you may remember
or have experienced it, dentistry consisted primarily of tooth pull-
ing. I remember as a child tying strings to loose teeth and thence

to a doorknob, then trying to slam the door. If a tooth was too stubborn for this approach, or if I wasn't able to do that final slam, consulting a dentist who had more powerful means of extraction was the way to go! The automobile ride into his office was a thing of dangling strings and nightmares.

We're talking about big-time pain, specifically associated with our teeth. Whether you were a child experiencing this or a parent watching, you could count on having to deal afterward with a swollen jaw or even an infected tooth. Dental phobia was well and fully instilled!

Now, remember the era: the Depression, with its all-pervading lack of funds. A few of you may also remember apples and pencils sold on the street or Roosevelt's mission to alleviate the worst of want with WPA and CCC work projects that hired thousands, along with the inception of social security benefits. Still, for most, even with these aids, money for dentistry came in poor second to money for food, shelter, and clothing.

Some of you may remember that, in an attempt to alleviate the cost of a visit to a dentist, providers would include wonderful smelling and tasting toothpastes. The proposal was: "Ipana for the smile of beauty; Sal Hepatica for the smile of health!" promulgating an affordable, if not long-term effective, dental and breath treatment. (And, for the liver, who knows?) The manufacturers did well—users of the products considerably less so.

Frequency of brushing counts! Fair is fair: brushing was, and is, certainly part of the answer to dental health, but only part!

There is one other event many children and, for that matter, adults went through in previous but remembered eras. If a tooth developed an increasingly painful cavity and it was in an easily seen part of the smile, an appointment was scheduled, trepidation notwithstanding, to "fix" it.

This fix, in turn, most likely created more dental phobia.

OFFICE AND INSTRUMENT ANXIETY

First, the setting for treatment was a hard-seated enamel armchair—like some variant of a barber's chair—that could be raised at the dentist's convenience but left the patient with a sense of doom and a kind of semi-airborne insecurity.

Next, by the side of this chair was a Rube Goldberg device consisting of several metallic joints and knobs through which cloth-wrapped wires stood ready to activate the point of a drill. The drill itself produced not only a loud, room-filling whine but also a painful, rotating burr as it excavated the tooth prior to the application of an amalgam filling. Any number of years later, this filling had to be redrilled, rereamed, and refilled with silver. The only analgesic on offer at these times was "spirit of clove" applied to the gum. I think many, like me, began to associate the medicine with tough torture and became frightened by its sight alone.

With the advent of WWII, a number of factors radically changed the institution of dentistry. A large population of military recruits in the army or navy were required to have dental treatments, rather than extractions, as GI standard care. Protocol for this included the use of novocaine as an inception. The changing standard of care became the idea of permanent repair or filling cavities as a standard approach to dental problems.

With the '50s came major tooth replacements with plates that were frequently mass-manufactured and therefore not infrequently ill-fitting. But as the '60s arrived, these became replaced by personal palate-measured and fitted devices.

DENTISTRY COMES OF AGE

The '80s and '90s brought tooth implants, again individualized patient by patient and installed painlessly with appropriate anesthesia (even with the additional humanity of proffered pre-procedure tranquilizers). Since then, more sophisticated and more quickly installed implant therapy has become the standard, together with cosmesis as a desirable and accepted norm.

More importantly, recognition and treatment has come to be critical to dental care. The recognition, superseding all of this development, relates to the more basic condition of the gum that holds the teeth, which needs both treatment and maintenance!

You may brush 'til the cows come home, but it doesn't substitute, or even partially erase, the critical importance of gum treatment. Which is why our gums have become perhaps the primary focus of dental care. If your gums aren't in a healthy state, dental replacement—rather than care—becomes the norm (not an entirely happy state of affairs).

Economically speaking, much of dentistry is now covered by medical insurance (not the cosmetic part, of course). The cost of that insurance is on a dealer's choice basis, or, in other words, it comes out of your own pocket.

Another consideration: today's crop of dentists are the product of two years of postgraduate university-based instruction before DDS can be attached to their names, and thereafter, many complete residencies in advanced or specialized dental techniques.

And, not atypically, today's dentist will examine the lymph nodes of the neck, inspect the entire mouth and tongue for signs of trouble, and suggest treatment for such entities as dry mouth or cold sores. All of this advancement should help to alleviate fears or concerns about dental care and encourage regular six-month visits to the dentist.

Now, having dealt with dental phobia and discussed the existence of healthy and aesthetic modern dental choices, there remains an even more important dental topic to address.

NUTRITION AND TEETH

I'm sure you are familiar with a well-known saying: "You are what you eat." It's a little shopworn, but as with so many old saws, its truth is enduring.

Let's look at two extreme illustrations. Consider that most of the people who were released from concentration camps as virtual skeletons were fed only a kind of attenuated potato soup not more than once a day. This was a diet meant to eliminate those no longer capable of working under the arduous camp conditions. Complete malnutrition. I learned this from a patient who needed a total hip replacement—it was part of his medical past.

And, on the other hand, with today's access to fast food and universal cola drinks, an overwhelming number of people face obesity. With increased rates of obesity have come an astronomical statistical rise in diabetes, early heart disease, and general physical decline that must be ascribed, in large part, to diet. Again, this is actually an example of malnutrition.

At age fifteen, or even twenty-five, you may get by with a diet of sweets and fast food. But when you are over sixty, nutrition becomes a subject to be taken and observed seriously, not quickly processed. To maintain general good health, a diet of protein (fish counts), essential minerals, vitamin-rich foods (usually undercooked vegetables or salads), and a bit of oil is an absolute requirement.

If your dentition is questionable or compromised, or if it hurts to eat meats (hamburger excepted), salad, or even some fruits (such as apples), you are going to be consuming a compromised diet that may well impair your nutrition. And your body will not accept this impairment for long. Thus, you may become subject to some elements of malnutrition, which, over any substantial period, will lead to seriously diminished health. This is why treatment for gingival (or gum) maintenance is considered *essential*.

So, our adage here becomes: take proper care of your teeth, and chances are, they will take care of you. Then, too, biting without hesitation into one thing or another may provide all kinds of enjoyment. And here's a parting thought: if you wish your adorable grandchild to offer that rosebud mouth rather than a quick-turned ear for a kiss, rendezvous regularly with your dentist.

Tend to your teeth, and they will tend to you!

WHOOPI'S TWO CENTS

You know, everybody says, "Get over your phobia of the dentist." But in these pandemic days, it's hard to know when any of us are next going to see a dentist. I mean really. Who's gonna lay there with their mouth open? I don't know who's going to do that.

But you know, find a dentist who will give you laughing gas. All you people who are stoic and say, "I'm going to do it without the gas," are ridiculous. Give me the drugs. Let me think I am at the Copacabana, and take out the teeth you need to take out. It's better for me, and it's better for the dentist. But again, you're not going to the dentist right now, so make sure you brush your teeth. Brush up and down and side to side in little circular motions. That's how you do it, okay? Make sure to brush your tongue, too, because there's nothing worse than someone with good breath and a horrifying tongue. Trust me.

PART FOUR
Broad Well-Being

Sometimes experience trumps assumption.

WHOOPI GOLDBERG

HOW TO TRAIN YOUR KEEPER

INACTIVITY: THE ENEMY

DON'T GET OUT OF BED SO SOON

SENIOR SKIN CARE

SPORTS AND PHYSICAL ACTIVITY

LIVING IN THE PAST

THE TIME I IGNORED MY OWN ADVICE

AFTER THE FALL

MEDICATIONS: TAKE FULL CONTROL

SELF-EXAMINATION (YES, I DO MEAN YOURS!)

How to
Train Your Keeper

DR. H

As we get older, get retired, or start receiving monthly social security checks or pensions, a change in human relations seems to occur between an Old Broad, her society, and her loved ones. This is particularly true if you've had some kind of major health problem, such as partially disabling arthritis, heart conditions, or trouble with memory.

Any of these problems may require the help of a part-time or even full-time caretaker. You may be in actual need of some help with things today that you did by rote for many years previously: changing clothes, preparing meals, banking, or shopping, to mention a few. Having good help can relieve you of frustration or anxiety when you may not be able to perform these simple or diurnal acts, much less those that take a bit more strength and vigor.

However, you must draw a sharp line between the tasks with which you're willing to accept help and those you consider precious "independencers." You need a no-go response before someone takes over your life! Here are some tips to help you avoid such a takeover:

- Be scrupulously honest in your assessment of where you are physically and/or mentally—what you really can do and what you have trouble with. If you're performing a certain task well enough, don't accept aid. If not, give in with good grace.
- Do not surrender—even to a loving family member— functions you know you can do for yourself, whether in the traditional way or using a work-around.
- Do not allow your family, in their attempts to love and care for you, go overboard in their efforts to protect you from anything they see as a hazard or too demanding.
- Work on your physical conditioning and enlarging your social circle via religious communities, neighborhood clubs, postings on your gated community bulletin board, or social app sites and groups. Do not let these activities be selected and moderated for you.
- Keep up with the world and the news of the day by reading articles on the internet or in a newspaper or watching television. This way, you will not need interpreters to explain the parlance of today.

At times you will find yourself in a "thank you, but no" position with respect to overzealous or oversolicitous help. Be sure in these moments to offer a big, "Thank you, but no," to the attempted takeover.

SOME SIMPLE STUFF

- Don't let others' overcaring rob you of putting on your own shoes. There is an easily available long-handled shoehorn that will permit you to accomplish this with ease.
- Don't give up on mobility when what you need is a walkerette.
- Don't rely on your keeper to fetch things for you when you could use a grabber to get those things on high shelves or at a distance.
- Continue making personal decisions, like choosing your clothing for the day. Your choice hasn't atrophied with age, nor has your opinion on planning your day. You're quite capable of doing it for yourself.

What you want to establish are basic ground rules: that you will ask for help when and if you need it, and if you don't, you don't! Acknowledge that you appreciate the intent beneath the unneeded help and appreciate the care that also underlies it but really prefer to do things for yourself when you can.

Here are some other how-tos:

- If necessary, stage a demonstration!
- You may have to repeat or reinforce your independent activity training (policy of anti–unneeded assistance) more than once.
- Don't get impatient, just train until it sticks.

I did all of the above when it came my turn to be "helped." But I also used personal intimidation, both verbal and facial. And you can, too, when it comes down to a specific situation. It's rare that I issue a complete verbal put-down, but I am known to use so-called "genius words" in English, German, French, or Latin that few people understand. Others don't have to know exactly what I'm saying to know they're on the receiving end of my temper.

When setting ground rules, I made sure my helper knew I was an egghead with three advanced degrees, one of them in medicine. I also used an extensive command of the King's English. In brief, I intimidated.

My ways were, looking back, a bit crude or unnecessarily dictatorial. But you get the underlying intent. There's always something you can use to intimidate or impress. Use it!

There are some words that ring true no matter the age, the language, the surroundings, or the source. We all know them, we all know how to act on them, but we sometimes overlook or disregard them at our own cost.

They are simply this: "You make the difference."

Inactivity: The Enemy

DR. H

I like to sit and watch TV, enjoy a must-read book, and sometimes just daydream awhile. But I know that, as happy as I am lying back in my favorite chair, when I'm doing so, I am being inactive. And if I let inactivity become a major part of my waking hours, well, I'm in all kinds of trouble.

Inactivity spawns a big-time disappearing act for your muscles and your shape. It rewards your arthritis with more pain. It encourages you to look to a bottle of pain relievers or anti-inflammatory meds for help, ignoring the source of trouble, which is disuse or inactivity.

As a result, you spend even more time dwelling on your pains and increasing stiffness while decreasing range of motion. Not a happy thing.

So, even though you may get bored with an exercise program, take my advice and move. As Whoop would say, "Just effing do it."

So much for the physical.

Next, let's talk about the mental. I'm a doctor, so, of course, I know the brain is not a muscle—even though I have referred to people of a certain personality type as muscle-heads. I also know that you still need to exercise your brain.

There are many ways to keeping the brain active. There are puzzle games of all sorts online or in print. Simply keeping up with what's happening in the world—via newspapers or journals or, least preferable, television news programs—is mental stimulation. And how about exchanging views with your friends or partner or grandkids? As to the last, don't be surprised at the new avenues of conversation they can come up with! Learning something new is, as I've often said, a kick in the head.

Social activity is also a great way to add spice to life. When you interact with others, you get to hear about both similar and different problems they're having with their families or learn about new books or articles that might interest you. You may even learn a new joke. I'm nuts for jokes. Here's one: Two olives scooch over to the end of a bar, and one falls off! The first olive yells to the olive on the floor, "Are you okay?" The olive on the floor responds, "Yes, I'm o-live!"

Sometimes things come up in your family or life that a good social acquaintance can help solve. Many times, sharing your scenario incites more conversation—a priceless experience.

But beware! Passive listening is a kind of inactivity where you're coasting along with someone else's ideas, way of life, or point of view without trying to assert your own. If you read an article or news report and simply swallow it whole, taking it in without any sort of question, you are being passive in the worst sense. Old Broads may not be able to add a great deal to our physiques, but we sure as hell should want to add to our armamentarium of ideas and information.

Not only for your sake but also for that of your near and dear, avoid the temptation to turn into an inactive—and therefore often repetitive—*bore*!

Oh. Wait, hold the phone! Here's a thought. We all have inhibitions, some left over from old mistakes or embarrassments. It's time you dropped these. They're the most negative form of "been there." If later experience hasn't conquered them, self-cure your inhibitions on the spot.

If I could wish just one thing for each of you, I would wish you a tiger's heart in your less-than-tiger body that impels you to be present and always be one of the active members of society.

WHOOPI'S TWO CENTS

Haha, sure! You can try anything. Supplements and running and jumping and exercising. People say, "Make sure you stretch when you get up." Okay, I will try that—not. I know I probably should exercise, but I'm not gonna do it.

I just spent some money on a Hula-Hoop; that Hula-Hoop is sitting there in the closet, gathering dust, because, even though in my mind I am an exercising fool, in reality—not so much. You know, I'll walk a little bit, I'll saunter a little bit, but you have to commit to all of those exercises.

I have friends who exercise like fiends, and they look terrific. I still look like a linebacker, but I'm me, so that's how I get past it. Every now and then I do think I should take some weight off. Then again, every now and then I think I should do a lot of things.

But what you should do is stretch when you wake up. I can hear Dr. Hecht right now saying, "Don't tell people not to stretch!" So yes, stretch when you wake up. And if you get to your toes by the time you're eighty, that's a fantastic thing. Up and down, stretch and touch your toes. Do your best. That's all you can do.

Don't Get Out of
Bed So Soon

DR. H

A s we grow older, many, if not most, of us develop some degree of arthritis (osteoarthritis) involving our major joints. This is most likely the result of the upright position that we humans have adopted, plus the additional stress we put on our bodies when we walk—or, particularly, as we run or jog—and the temporal consequence of age. But it's unavoidable, as we probably won't go back to the apelike four-limb ambulation that would prevent many problems pursuant to uprightness. (I mean what would the neighbors think?)

Our bodies announce or demonstrate arthritis with symptoms of stiffness and pain, especially in the early morning hours. Actually, even after a successful joint replacement, you may still experience some early morning symptoms. But your aching bones, emphatically, should not be the first thing on your mind as you start your day. Let that be at least something like: *My favorite program is on TV today!* or *My favorite niece is coming to call!* or even maybe *It's Sunday; I'll have waffles for breakfast!*

Whether you have undergone joint replacement surgery or are just beginning to acquire beginning arthritic twinges, there is something positive you can do to modify your arising state and rid yourself of the boy-do-I-ache blues. No, it doesn't require anti-inflammatory meds, massage, heat, and/or physical therapy—any and all of which may also modify your pain, stiffness, and some degree of disability.

What I want you to do before you decide what kind of day it's going to be—even as you open your eyes—is a series of bed exercises. With these or any other exercise, always inhale to begin, then exhale on execution. This will help with your breathing along the way! Also, do not hold your breath while doing any exercise.

Let's get started.

BREATHING EXERCISE

Position: Lie flat on your back in bed.

1. If you are a side or stomach sleeper, roll onto your back.
2. Take in as deep a breath as you can, always through your nose.
3. Hold it for a count of five.
4. Then slowly blow out as much air as you can. Every bit of it! Always through your mouth.
5. Repeat five times.
6. Though I start the day with this exercise, you can sit down and go through it anytime you feel breathless or short of breath. It works like a charm.

WAKE UP YOUR SPINE

———

Position: Lie flat on your back in bed.

1. Slowly bend one knee until you can grasp it with both hands, assisting it up as near as you can to your stomach.
2. Hold it there for a slow count of ten.
3. Then, gradually, release the knee and let it return to its original position.
4. Do the same with the other leg.
5. Next, grasp both knees, and bring them up to your chest.
6. Hold the position for a count of twenty.
7. Work up gradually until you can do a minimum of five repetitions.

Check what this simple exercise will do for your mobility and as a pain-lessening tool.

SHOULDER MOTION

———

Position: Lie flat on your back in bed.

1. Start with your arms straight at your sides, then raise them slowly, aiming to go toward the side of your head.
2. Continue the upward motion as far as you can reach above your head.
3. Repeat five times.

ANKLES NEXT

—

Position: Lie flat on your back in bed.

1. Pump both ankles up and down gently, slowly, going as far as you can.
2. Do at least twenty repetitions.

SIT UP

—

Position: Sit up (slowly) on the side of your bed.

1. Gently shrug your shoulders five times.
2. Next, raise your arms as high as you can, then drop them to your sides slowly. Repeat five times.

LEGS

—

Position: Sit on the side of your bed with your feet on the floor.

1. Slowly extend and straighten each knee as far as you can without pain.
2. Return to the seated position with your knees bent.
3. Repeat five times initially, working toward ten and then twenty repetitions over time.

NECK

Position: Sit on the side of your bed with your feet on the floor.

1. Drop your chin to your chest, then raise it gently and slowly toward the ceiling. Repeat five times.
2. Drop your head to your chest and roll it slowly side to side (ear to chest to ear). Repeat five times.
3. Try to look as far as you can to the right, then to the left. Repeat five times.

THE FINALE!

Position: Rise from your bed. Then go back to bed and start the entire series again.

Of my patients who tried this lie-in-bed-and-wake-up-slowly routine, nearly all reported it was of real help. When you think about its intent and what is reasonable—a relatively short transition from the comfort of your blankets to being up and about—this series is clear, concise, and effective.

ADDITIONAL TIPS

- You may not be able to do these limber-up exercises with full motion due to joint stiffness, a large tummy, and so on. Don't worry; do the best you can within the range possible.
- Chances are if these exercises help, you'll do them regularly. But if you have a so-so result, do them

when you can. Skipping a day or two won't ablate their benefit.

- Remember to breathe in with each movement and out on the excursion. I don't want you getting short of breath.
- Don't abandon the practice if you miss a session or two; as the saying goes, all is grist that comes to the mill. And all of us Old Broads are at least part grist as opposed to muscle.

So then, off you go!

Senior Skin Care

DR. H

I f it hasn't for one reason or another been a priority, or longtime responsibility, the care and pleasure of body maintenance as you enter your sixty-plus years should be of prime importance.

I mean, rather than change the TV channel when appearance-enhancing commercials are on, or even programs where you begin to think what you can do to make your years disappear, and promise you'll look if not pampered, at least well cared for. Not just your face, but your entire persona. If you're smart you won't see these as real care, but, by and large, promos of product marketing.

Real senior body care takes some doing and extra focus but will repay you in terms of the respectful attention you'll receive, your sense of well-being, or even plain out loud admiration. It is achievable, but does take time, practice, and consistent focus.

Don't despair if you see only the wrinkles and crags on the face that greets you come morning. A major factor in senior skin care is simply that: care. For example, did you know that the universal age phenomenon of wrinkles is partially caused by a lack of water? There is no way that the freshness of youthful skin can be duplicated by drinking water. But you also never have to accept totally withered or ashen skin—or, for that matter, such an age phenomenon as whiskers (inappropriate facial hair growth).

About water: One thing you can do to help get more water to your skin is apply a simple cream containing major hyaluronic acid. The key here—in addition to the essential element of hyaluronic acid—is the recognition that applying this once, when you get up in the morning, isn't sufficient. Doing so midday and again at night does the trick. It's the rule of consistency or regularity of application!

Regarding the matter of Botox products: Yes, they do help (by paralyzing the facial muscles). But the medical jury is out on how many times it's advisable to receive Botox injections. The period of effectiveness for each injection is most often cited at around six months.

Also, plumping up facial areas that are "creased" with JUVÉDERM or other fillers can be done; but again, how many times it should be repeated is the question.

About facial hair: Shaving or razing may actually increase its stubbornness and consistency. Plucking or waxing is probably the way to go. These methods must be repeated at intervals of recurrence but can be done safely. Be careful of things that look like pencils but are actually razors. They tend to do the job but seem to require more and more frequent application and are, in essence, electric shavers. Remember that toes and fingers also require regular attention.

About soaps and shampoos: The safest in terms of avoiding an allergic response are still the simple, perfume-free, additive-free soaps. And shampoos created for babies are great if they do the job.

About body coverings (e.g., dress, nightwear, coats, etc.): Natural fabrics are better for your skin than substitutes (e.g., Dacron, various acetates, nylon, etc.). Gloves are a good idea in all seasons. Net gloves for summer help to prevent contact with harmful substances. And come winter, if your hands aren't warm, the rest of you shivers. Consider warmth as an essential part of choosing appropriate dress—whether you're at home or out. And, in light of the COVID-19 pandemic, wash hands frequently, and don't touch new or unknown surfaces without gloves.

IN GENERAL

You are best off completing a daily overall inspection for such things as new growths, color changes, or blemishes anywhere on your body or anything you feel was not present before. I'm tempted to say, like brushing your teeth, it should be a routine you always complete before going out in public or meeting with others. Also, little seeming growths or changes in pigmentation may tip you off as an early sign of malignancy. If caught and treated at this early stage, they're often completely treatable.

Try not to go through your day with anything that causes discomfort, like a dress or slacks being too tight or shoes that cause pinching. Fit is as important as function and appearance. And discomfort may lead to longer-term irritation.

There may be other entirely individual or special factors that you, as the owner of your body, will best be able to identify and ameliorate. Perhaps you have a frozen joint and need to rethink zippers, or maybe you deal with Raynaud's syndrome and need warmer gloves year-round. Whatever it is, don't ignore it. Attend to it with care at the moment it's perceived!

What this topic of senior skin care comes down to is that, as we grow into seniority, things may need particular attention regularly. Your body needs age-appropriate and consistent inspection and care. It's a basic of well-being. It's also a matter of being smart.

Even though you may need some help from others ("Can you hold the mirror so I can see the back?"), remember, you're the CEO of your own body. So behave like one!

Sports and Physical Activity

DR. H

I've gotten a lot of questions from patients about the kind of physical activity that is most helpful after the age of sixty. So here's some of the advice I have given to them.

My first bit of advice is: *be patient, and don't take chances.* Think ahead before you do anything new or different. This may sound like advice from an overprotective mother hen, but I assure you, it's not.

The two forms of exercise that I am a big fan of are fast walking and swimming. I love the pool as it makes us weightless and affords us a great protected workout. And I advise you to fast walk as much as you like once your doctor gives you the go-ahead and you have passed your physical.

But there are also always new sports to try. Perhaps you never gave golf a shot. I want to tell you, it's a fascinating sport. And for those of you in the know, Jack Nicklaus and Arnold Palmer both golfed well into their seventies with total hip replacements!

Even so, remember: safe, not sorry! Before you start new athletic activities for the first time, it's not a bad thought to check with your doctor. The bottom line is whatever your chosen activity is, just keep moving! Take responsibility for your fitness and health, and you'll maximize your sixties, seventies, and beyond.

There are three types of exercise that you need to maintain your general physical well-being. They are:

1. Aerobic (AER)—most often thought of as cardiorespiratory conditioning
2. Toning (TON)—involves building strength and muscular endurance
3. Range of motion (ROM)—a self-explanatory phrase referring to the use of all your joints
4. A combination of all three is what we call general conditioning (GENCON)

Interest, convenience, availability, and which of these three types is most needed for you will dictate which sport(s) you do. One sport may contain more of one type than another. Ideally, you'd get a little of all three types.

SWIMMING

Swimming is great for aerobic and range of motion. A YMCA, health club, or pool can usually be found not too far away. Classes in aquatic exercises are a top option for GENCON. I particularly like aqua-aerobic classes because you're weightless in water and can't damage arthritic knees, ankles, and hips.

PELOTON CYCLING
AND ROWING MACHINES

Peloton cycling is the latest version of spinning with the added excitement of virtual classes, music, and instructors. The home exercise bike has a large video screen that connects you to live and on-demand aerobic workouts. Rowing machines offer a great general conditioning body workout simulating crewing or rowing on a river. Watch out for kids near the machine—they can get in trouble.

YOGA

Age-appropriate yoga, and especially chair yoga (where a high-back chair serves as a barre), is superb for range of motion. It's also a good breathing workout. Hot yoga is also good for general conditioning.

TENNIS

This popular sport is great for general conditioning. The social side is fun too. And it's available all season, as there are so many indoor courts.

GOLF

This general conditioning workout offers great scenery and is a great competitive group sport. Also, there's always the nineteenth hole to quench the thirst your group has worked up. Golfers can be seen playing well into their eighties or even nineties thanks to the ubiquity of golf carts.

BOXING

Boxing has many benefits for us over sixty, including just being fun. The newest trend, "fitness boxing," involves tossing punches at a bag for a general conditioning workout—and the best part is, this comes without the risk of someone hitting you back. It helps strengthen your core, back, shoulders, arms, and leg muscles (toning) while increasing flexibility (range of motion).

FAST WALKING

This is a perfect aerobic and general conditioning exercise. But while I'm on the subject, as an orthopedic surgeon, I don't recommend jogging or running unless you want to support someone's orthopedic practice. Running and/or jogging result, more frequently than not, in the need for early knee or even hip replacement.

BOWLING

Bowling is good for toning as long as your back and knees are okay. But even so, it's an amusement rather than a sport. But it comes with lots of bragging rights when you hit a number of strikes.

THE TOPIC OF FITNESS CENTERS

Best to pick and choose very carefully here because many trainers encourage too much resistance (too heavy weights) and put you through the paces too quickly if you are not already working out (injuries waiting to happen).

Remember, bragging rights have no place when you're working with weights or increased resistance. It's fitness you're after, not an Arnold Schwarzenegger or Charles Atlas look. Pride (your ego) may also lead to overestimation. Weight lifting then may well cause injury rather than toning, shaping, or strengthening.

With apologies to those trainers who have studied anatomy and physiology, the weights and kettlebells many propose may inadvertently cause injury, and those of us over sixty are especially vulnerable. It's true that there is a wide variety of conditioning that lets some do what others can't. Just remember to be open-minded in the perception of what is safe for you.

PROCEED WITH CAUTION
AND ENTHUSIASM

I hope I have mentioned some of the major or most practiced sports and fitness options. I wrote this piece because, as a physician, I strongly believe in the fundamental importance of physical activity. One mantra I am not a fan of is the "no pain, no gain" formula, which only asks for big-time trouble!

Physical activity, exercise, and sports in the life of seniors, especially as they age, is a must. Here, the legitimate mantra of "use it or lose it" fits!

There is, as always, enjoyment in sports and physical activity. Be sure to adjust your choice of sport and your level expectation from when you may have participated in your twenties and thirties. And enjoy the fact that you can participate well into your nineties— *admired by all.*

My final two cents: exercise is fun for some, but, aside from golf, it was not always my cup of tea. Therefore, I would bring along an exercise buddy and treat some of these sports as social occasions to help me get through. So extra brownie points if you induce company to share all the physical and social benefits.

Living in the Past

DR. H

I had a completely self-absorbed career back in my theater days, and I made no effort to make deep friends. Instead, I acquired many colleagues who shared my interests and preoccupations. Back then the world was my oyster, and I had little care for what might be problems or difficulties for others. When a colleague became in the least boring or in any way troublesome, I simply abandoned their company.

Talk about the great disposable society. I was primo; a party animal par excellence. We all know how significant and lasting parties are.

It wasn't until I went through medical school and took the Hippocratic oath (the heart of which is "above all, do no harm") that I began to become empathetic and to have a sense of responsibility for my fellow humans. We all can look back at the people we once were and wallow in regrets. Please don't.

Too much rehearsing or dwelling at length over what's happened in the past is a no-no for Old Broads unless the visitation to the past is:

- colorful
- humorous
- a onetime trip
- slightly salacious or even risqué

But be sure it is!

Dwelling on age, aches, and pains or "things I can't do anymore" is off-limits! Strictly off-limits!

I have on occasion excused myself from conversations and finally tried the self-indulgence of absence to another room (a move that's in the sly fox but slightly antisocial department). But if you want to contribute something to an ongoing conversation without dwelling on the past, you can never go wrong with these tips:

1. *Stay current.* Show some interest in someone else's day or happenings. Consider interest as a two-way street. Also try talking about current events.
2. *Be selfless.* Make a point of asking about and listening to the problems of others, and, if asked, offer possible answers or solutions or reference sources.
3. *Humor.* Bring it on! Try to cultivate and share with others. (I don't mean Joe Miller jokes, but shaggy dog humor often makes a favorable ripple in encounters.)

I think you get the idea.

I also think you'll get a kick out of the results.

Now that I'm over ninety and have practiced the things I've written about here for a number of years, I can only continue to practice what I preach and thank the powers that be for the opportunity to do so.

The Time I Ignored My Own Advice

DR. H

In my early seventies I was late for a dinner date with a friend in NYC. The light was typical of winter at seven o'clock. I was hurrying along, my thoughts on the ticking clock and the inconvenience I was causing my friend. Then, before I knew it, I was upside down on the ground. I had completely missed a broken curb and went head over heels into a fall onto my right hip.

I knew, of course, by the immediate pain and inability to freely move my leg that I had fractured it. The diagnosis was not difficult for an orthopedist, but the knowledge that I had ignored my own safeguarding advice was a mixture of mind-blowing, humiliating, and rage-inducing.

Yes, there were crowds around me. But in the Big Apple there is often a reluctance to get involved with any kind of accident because you might become an unwilling part of it. When I got over my fury with myself, retrieved my phone, and called 911, I stayed exactly where I'd fallen. Better the cold ground than risking a displacement of a fracture or causing additional bleeding.

What should I have done to avoid all this? Followed my Three-Look Method of moving through the world with safety.

THE THREE-LOOK METHOD

Think of the times you've gotten in trouble or even hurt. Isn't it possible you've said to yourself, "If I'd only looked to see . . ." or "If I'd only listened for . . ." or "If I'd only taken my time . . ."?

But how do you teach yourself to do these things consistently?

To teach yourself any new thing, you must master or remember it by constant and deliberate repetition. If you're one who never goes to sleep without an evening prayer, make these simple words, in effect, your morning invocation: *stop, listen,* and *look.*

> *First:* Stop (or pause) for a moment before entering new or unfamiliar surroundings.
>
> *Second:* Listen for any strange or warning sounds.
>
> *Third:* Look, look, and look again. I don't mean a glance or a peek. Really look! Use the deliberate Three-Look Method to protect yourself in any circumstance. It goes like this:

> *Step 1:* *Look low*—at the floor or street level.
>
> *Step 2:* *Look level*—at chairs or midpoint objects in your way. Look both left and right.
>
> *Step 3:* *Look up*—toward the ceiling or sky.

Practice the Three-Look Method over and over, and do it consistently whether you're in a familiar or brand-new environment.

It may seem a lot to think about. But actually, as an invocation, it can become a new habit that helps you each and every night and day. As you use it more and more, it will get both easier and more effective.

Having once so disastrously ignored this advice, I do follow my own program. So, to reiterate: stop, listen, and look three times. You may avoid an event both you and your dear ones wish to never happen.

Here are some possible add-on tips to help you avoid trouble:

- *Anticipate.* If you're ready to go somewhere or do something, particularly if it is not familiar, think about what could be difficult or problematic. Think before you leap—or even hop!
- *Use your brain at all times.* Don't do anything on automatic pilot. As much as possible, stay alert and in an anticipatory mode during all waking hours, whether you're at home or in public. As the kids might say, stay "in the moment" and "check it all out."
- *Don't be embarrassed to ask for help.* Most people love to feel helpful. It may become the high point in a day that's routine—or even become good cocktail or dinner talk. Can you hear it? "I helped this elderly woman up into the bus," or "I made sure this elderly gent crossed the road safely." Good Samaritans earn what we used to call brownie points and the regard of their peers. So don't be embarrassed to ask for or accept help!
- *Be safe, not sorry.* If there are two known ways to get somewhere or do something, choose the way you know is safe rather than the one that is quicker or nearer.
- *Stop rushing.* It's one of the most consistent and hazardous mistakes for older citizens! It causes trips and falls,

obviates care and self-protection, encourages mindless activity, and almost always leads to trouble.

Here's what it comes down to: forewarned is forearmed, which is a really desirable condition.

After the Fall

DR. H

write this chapter as an author, patient, and idiot! The Three-Look Method is in no way a wiseacre's do-what-I-say, not-what-I-do advice. In my own defense, we all have our little lapses.

Once the EMTs got me onto a gurney, I persuaded them to take me to Cabrini Medical Center in NYC where I practiced at the time. When we arrived, the ER personnel were more than familiar with me, so they acceded to two requests. First, they performed an immediate X-ray of my hip, and second, they contacted one of my orthopedic colleagues to take charge of what I knew would be surgery. Obviously, I had an advantage in this situation that few others do, but hey, it made me feel better to give orders when I knew I would have to take a great many more from others after my inevitable surgery.

When Dr. Perle arrived, we reviewed the X-ray together. Dr. Perle had been my student during his hospital residency, and despite my best effort to inculcate good bedside manners to all my clinical orthopedic residents, the man had none whatsoever. As a matter of fact, he had a huge ego, but this deficit was earned by the fact that he was one of the most skillful orthopedic surgeons I had ever worked with. Exactly what I wished for in the situation of my affected hip.

The X-rays showed not one but two severely arthritic hips, one of which was embellished with a fracture. Dr. Perle said, "We'll do the fractured right hip tomorrow and the left a few weeks later."

No! I wrapped myself in the mantle of the senior orthopedist and commanded, "We'll do one side, then flip me over and do the other." And that's exactly what he did.

Despite my stupidity in evoking the injury, I grant that I had some advantages in this situation: a hospital where I'd been on staff that gave me preferred status to receive an early surgery; a nursing and technical staff that handled one of their own with kid gloves; immediate attention; my choice of surgeon; and a private room.

Within four weeks I was back in my own orthopedic practice booking arthroscopic procedures, which allow you to sit while performing them rather than standing at the side of an operating table.

An afterthought leads me to add that my recovery included considerable pain, tough physical therapy sessions, and some social limitations. Perhaps worse was a certain chagrin at having ignored the advice I gave to all my patients about the Three-Look Method.

As an Old Broad you should no longer assume that hazards don't lie within the familiar places of your home or any place you've deemed safe and sound. Think about how often you've heard someone who was injured "in my own house" or "on my own front porch" say something like, "I don't understand; I was just walking into my hallway when—boom!"

SO YOU'VE FALLEN!

It's easy to panic, but you must doublethink. Fear and/or panic will not help! Instead, follow these three steps:

Step 1: *Free your mouth of any impediment*—such as the rug or carpet if you're in a facedown position, covers, etc.—and take several deep, slow breaths. Try to call 911. I hope, as I've advised my patients to do, you are wearing a medical-alert device for just such a purpose.

Step 2: *Try to avoid panic.* First, use your knowledge of where you are and your perceived state to relate information in the call for help. "Help, I've fallen, and my hip, my back, or my wrist is very painful." If you're wise, you'll have your critical medical and personal information list on hand.

Step 3: *Don't try to rise.* Remember, I followed this step on the Manhattan sidewalk. Wait for help. You may add to harm with an unsuccessful attempt to get up.

Again, make a conscious effort not to let fear or anxiety take over. At a time like this, the clock seems never to move, but it always does.

If you managed most of the above, bravo! You've contributed substantially to your chances of complete recovery and demonstrated the smartest and most impressive you.

Medications: Take Full Control

DR. H

At our age, daily medications are a given. Yesterday I talked to a friend in the well-over-sixty group. Medications came up because she was having what seemed to be side effects to one of her prescribed medications. I wondered if it was a new prescription that wasn't working with her existing ones. What I learned is that she couldn't tell because she had thrown all her medications in her bag without a system for identifying which one(s) should be taken at what time(s).

Fortunately, the side effect was nausea, which ceased when the misuse was clarified. I felt she was damn lucky that she didn't get into more trouble with a much more serious reaction.

The more she talked, the more I realized she wasn't on top of what she was taking and why. This disturbed me to no end and, at the same time, made me really sad. I hope it saddens you, too, because it should never happen!

I thought perhaps her confusion was due in part to short-term memory loss, plus embarrassment at having to ask her physician to explain in words of one syllable what was for what and when.

I was deliberately curt—even condescending—in my reproach over her lack of awareness of what meds she was taking and that she had not worked out a personal foolproof system for taking them at the right time. I mean curt to the point of using the word "stupidity."

A haphazard approach to meds at our age is an invitation for nothing but trouble. So here are some tips to help you expand your knowledge.

WHAT IS THE PILL AND WHAT DOES IT DO?

The chemical names on each prescription may not do much to reveal their value or use. Usually, the more familiar trade names are in small print at the bottom of the labels. But if neither name on a prescription rings a bell, ask your pharmacist what it's for. Don't get in the unenviable position of ingesting a pill or tablet without knowing precisely why you're using it. Use your handy marker pen to label each bottle. And be sure you know the expiration date.

To ensure that your meds are taken properly, you could either make a chart that you check daily and place in a visible location (like just beside the vials of medication or in the medications bag or box) or use one of those organizing plastic containers from the pharmacy. The best ones are divided into columns by days of the week and then divided into rows for each morning, midday, and evening. Fill it up! Then you never have to worry if you took a med or not. Though, of course, at the beginning of the week you have to load your container. This is one of those small gimmicks that is worth its weight in gold.

Having accounted for the everyday meds, be sure to list those meds needed for special circumstances—for example, nitroglycerine for chest pain or an antihistamine for minor allergic reactions—and know where you can get your hands on them immediately.

REORDER!

As you near the end of your box, or simply on a given day (Thursday, for example) toward the end of each month, call your pharmacist and/or arrange to pick up your supply for the next month. Either underline this date on your medication list or put a dot with fingernail polish or a marker pen on the appropriate day in the set of pill boxes.

DO YOU KNOW THE POTENTIAL SIDE EFFECTS?

Every prescription is required to list all possible side effects. So, if you have a magnifying glass handy and lots of patience, these are all to be found on the accompanying folded document, written, of course, in flyspeck.

If you go online and visit, say, Wikipedia or Google, the major side effects are easily discernible. Chances are your MD may also have given you a "look out for these major possible untoward side effects" talk when prescribing the medication. If you followed the Four Ears, One Notepad system, all the better.

HOW HAVE THE MEDS BEEN ORGANIZED (AND WHERE ARE THEY KEPT)?

This seems like a simple question, but daily administration is so critical that it may be best to choose one location—say, the table by your bed, the kitchen table, or the breakfast counter—that is to be the never-changing location of your pills and your list or weekly plastic meds container.

If you need injectables, perhaps select the bathroom where topical alcohol is available and your hypo and needles can be safe from little hands.

And if you have any signs of short-term memory deficits—and I do mean any (be honest here)—I strongly suggest you get a second pair of eyes to lay out and organize your meds week by week. This may sound namby-pamby until the first time you cannot, with certainty, remember whether or not you've taken an important medication.

YEARLY CHECK-INS WITH YOUR MD?

This is so obvious that I hesitate to mention it, but this event should be scheduled and listed as a to-do on an anniversary basis, unless any problem comes up before this yearly event.

WHAT IF YOU HAVE A REACTION?

An oddball side reaction can happen even with a medication you've been taking for months or years. As an MD I'm never surprised when a patient reports this. I haven't got a succinct answer as to why reactions happen. But consider this: every cell in your body is replaced every seven years. And the replacement, although almost alike in terms of function or anatomy or importance, is not identical. Your body cells at sixty have completely erased those you had at twenty and forty, so it is possible that they don't react or act in the identical way. If you question this, look in the mirror. The image staring back is recognizably you, miracle of miracle, but it's a totally different you.

If you have any odd reaction to a given medication, call your MD immediately. A substitute med can be prescribed. If you have a major untoward reaction—difficulty breathing, hives, or swelling about the mouth—you or your caregiver should be on the phone with the nearest emergency room for advice. If, for some reason, you're not able to get in touch with someone immediately, call 911!

WHO ELSE KNOWS?

Someone in the family or your caregiver should know exactly what you're taking, for what reason, and how it's to be taken. Most MDs advise those over sixty to carry a list of all their meds and the dosages they're taking. Why? Because that way, if there is an emergency, you don't have to remember all that info! Or, heaven forbid, you arrive in an emergency room unconscious or unable to articulate information.

Even more important is a list of allergies. For example, you may be allergic to one of the penicillin family (actually not uncommon), which are among the first line drugs used to help treat serious wounds. If you required emergency medical attention and your allergy was not known, the result would be catastrophic! I strongly suggest this list also be kept on your person; it could be written into a necklace, carried like an ID card, kept in your phone, and so on.

DO YOU USE THE SAME PHARMACY?

You should use the same pharmacy for all your prescriptions. They will keep a record of your medications and when renewals are ready. They will also tell you when your physician has to renew or even add to your retained list.

MEDICATIONS FROM ONLINE OR ABROAD?

There is the possibility of using a Canadian source for any drug advised by your MD that is not on the list covered by your insurance. You can find these online too. This is an option you positively must discuss with your MD. But Canadian drugs are cheaper than their American-made counterparts and easily shipped.

OPIATES?

The issue of opiates has been beaten to death by the press and, unfortunately, often comes to us in numbers of those who abuse and inappropriately dispense them. Then there are the stories of those who don't survive use, abuse, and availability. Remember that in your sixties you get more—not less—sensitive to many opiates. So be honest with yourself about these types of meds.

What I want to say is simple: if you need non-opioid painkillers, such as Aspirin, TYLENOL, Advil, and so on, keep them in the house to help with those difficult days or nights as needed. Also, opiates and age don't always go well together. A twenty-year-old may be able to use a med such as TYLENOL with Codeine No. 4 (containing three hundred milligrams of Codeine) with impunity, but as you get older, the amount of opiate (Codeine) may be too much for you. You may be able to get pain relief with TYLENOL with Codeine No. 2.

The side effects of almost any opiate can be dizziness, unsteadiness, blurred vision, and more. None of these should be visited upon you as a senior. If they are, report your experience to your MD as soon as possible. Be sure you isolate opioids from your regularly taken meds.

WHAT ABOUT SUPPLEMENTS?

The vitamin/mineral supplement business is a multitrillion-dollar industry. Before you spend your money, check with your MD that a given vitamin or mineral preparation would be appropriate for you.

Many preparations widely advertised may not be required or even helpful. When you take an excess of water-soluble (vitamins B and C) vitamins, they are eliminated by the kidneys. So, even if you overuse them, they are not likely to produce problems. However, fat- or oil-soluble (vitamins A or D) vitamins are handled by the liver and can actually become harmful if taken in large quantities. The body cannot so easily handle them.

Then there are over-the-counter preparations that promise the world: ablation of short-term memory loss, help for impotence, an increased sex drive, quick weight loss, and so on. These should be looked at askance. A phone call to your physician will give you a quick thumbs-up or thumbs-down opinion. Talk about smart!

LET YOUR MD BE
YOUR TRUE HEALTH PARTNER

———

In any case, be absolutely sure your MD knows what you take. Use telemedicine for quick and to-the-point conversations if need be.

Finally, it behooves us to remember that tiny hands have a way of getting into all sorts of things that are "childproof." So, if little hands are coming for a visit (or to stay), be sure your meds and/or their containers are on high, unladdered shelves or out of sight.

If you handle your meds in this or a similarly organized way, your near and dear will feel they can take one more concern off their list.

Self-Examination
(Yes, I Do Mean Yours!)

DR. H

When I submitted the first draft of this manuscript, my editor questioned the need for this chapter. "There's a whole month of the year dedicated to breast cancer awareness," she said. "Office complexes are festooned in pink ribbons, and housing developments turn their fountains pink. There are fundraisers and health screenings from coast to coast. Doesn't everyone know they need to examine their breasts by now?"

So I did a little surveying in the halls and elevators of my condo and found that breast health was not a part of one woman's self-care regimen.

Ha! Point proven.

If I were to ride through your town, city, or apartment building on a scooter wearing nothing but a tea cozy or a Red Sox baseball cap, I think you'd pay attention. And even though that won't be possible, I need your attention on this topic, so I'm sitting in the nude while writing this quintessential chapter. I want you to read it word for word—from beginning to end. I hope the image of a nude ninety-two-year-old typing away on her keyboard to promote the cause of self-examination stirs some interest in this chapter.

I think many of us don't want to hear much about—call it breast health—because we all are aware that breast cancer is the leading cause of cancer mortality for the female population. Also, many women think their breasts are the most feminine allurement they have. Treatment of the breast, however minimal, does leave its imprint and may lead to ablation (usually complete loss); therefore, this has become a feared and too often put-off topic.

However, breast cancer, with the exception of vicious cell types, is often beatable when caught early.

But if not treated early, your medical team has to play catch-up, and you'll be really lucky if they are able to do so entirely.

As an intelligent and with-it woman, you want to give early self-examination a go because:

- Breast cancer is most common in women between the ages of forty and seventy but may occur in your thirties or, in some cases, even earlier.
- It tends to run in the family.
- Obesity and early onset menstruation seem to be correlated with increased incidence of breast cancer.
- Breast cancer tends to occur undetected in heavy or dense breasts where physical examination is more difficult.
- Advanced cases of breast cancer may occur even without pain.
- Most irregularities, including lumps, aren't malignant or even premalignant. But they should be examined by an MD before being given this designation.

If you're afraid of what you may find and put off self-examination, a reluctant examination once a year is simply a kind of lip service to the problem. It is not remotely sufficient no matter what your fear! Once a month is a must. And you should do this examination with an open mind, as if you're performing it for the first time.

Are you thinking, *Well, I'm not a medical expert, so the next time I go to my gynecologist, I'll let her do the exam?* Let's face it: you don't actually go to your gynecologist or physician more than once a year. Cancer can strike the day after your last office visit.

I think I've made my point. So let's get to the physical technique and details.

BREAST EXAMINATION

There are many breast self-examination techniques. I'm going to share mine. But I must insist you check your method with your MD or gynecologist!

My Exam: I start by checking for any anomalies on the breast. Here's how:

- First, look for any dimpling or general shape irregularities.
- Then check for an inverted nipple (rare, but it needs investigation).
- Finally, check for a crusty sore spot.

Next, you want to examine all four quadrants of the breast: bottom left, bottom right, top left, and top right. To do this, move your breast away from the area you must palpate (feel), hold it steady with the opposite hand, and feel for any irregularities of texture or any lumps, however small. Follow these tips:

- Take your time to use your fingers to feel deep into the quadrant. Repeat several times.
- Palpate your axilla (armpit) for any nodes.
- If you encounter the smallest irregularity, do not panic. Many, if not most, slight differences in texture in the breast are normal, and many small nodes or lumps are also. But take note, reexamine the next day, and if your findings are the same, make a call to your gynecologist or MD, who will schedule a visit and then a mammogram. Mammographic examinations, as you must be aware, are the gold standard approach to confirmation of the physical exam of the breast.

Now, if you go through months or years of negative self-examination results, this is par for the course. Between the ages of forty and seventy, you should schedule a mammogram every year. You could do a mother-and-daughter mammogram day. The buddy system and company may be reassuring as opposed to a solo visit. Think of the treat you'll get after the exam: a martini, tea, cocoa, a martini—whatever's your favorite tipple.

Now, before you leave this chapter, how about the man in the household? He should be pursuing an exam for common and curable prostate problems. He probably can't do an appropriate self-exam, but if he shows signs of difficulty in urination or many night trips to the bathroom, he needs to go to his MD for an exam. For women, breast cancer is the common occurring cancer; for men, it's prostate cancer. Think of this parallel awareness as his and hers preventive medicine!

The whole issue of breast examination stirs in many of us a fear—you could almost say terror—of both the known and unknown consequences of a positive result.

I cannot tell you not to be fearful. But fear of the unknown and its possibility is even worse than fear of the known. The known implies a degree of control and even complete treatment.

Trust in this: most breast cancer, if caught early, is entirely curable. I only wish lung cancer from smoking were as treatable.

PART FIVE
Broad Shoulders

In the dark times, if you have something to hold on to,
which is yourself, you'll survive.

WHOOPI GOLDBERG

AM I LOSING MY MIND?

NODDING OFF

AN APPROACH TO YOUR WILL

LET'S TALK ABOUT ATTRITION

BREAKING MEDICAL NEWS

CROTCHETY WITH CHARM

Am I Losing My Mind?

DR. H

The terms "Alzheimer's" and "dementia" are sometimes used interchangeably. However, they refer to two radically different things: dementia is more a syndrome (group of symptoms), while Alzheimer's is a specific disease that could cost you your life.

Short-term memory loss is a damn inconvenience, but you are not really ill with it. The joke that someone can recite the first five amendments of the Constitution, or the "General Prologue" of Chaucer's *The Canterbury Tales*, but can't remember what they ate for breakfast this morning—defines short-term memory loss.

Lapses in short-term memory can produce unparalleled moments of panic and induce tears of fear. Many of us wonder if the can't-find-the-word-or-number episode is a one-off happening or the beginning of dementia. Natural enough. You may sit and recite your social security numbers or your zip code over and over just to reassure yourself that you can and vow to write them down on a card or pad that you will always carry on your person. Take heart.

This may mean nothing if you have never watched the game show *Jeopardy!*. I am a competitive *Jeopardy!* watcher whose scores range from less than 1900 to a record of several thousands, yet some days I can't remember anything in a whole category.

At some point you will wonder whether to share your memory lapses with your near and dear. Or you may think, *I can't tell my family; they'll freak out. Could it be a side effect of one of the meds I take?* The nights of worry can become endless.

Take it from Dr. Old Broad, if your memory lapse has manifested as an occasional one or two instances (and there's no reason or rhyme to when and what subject), wait a minute (or five!) before sharing the experience with someone who might lose sleep along with you. Don't think, *Dear God, am I getting Alzheimer's?* Take a breath, and turn to some other activity or focus your attention elsewhere. Nine times out of ten, within several minutes, the misplaced word or number will pop up in your mind. Isn't that a winning statistic?

If a day or a week goes by and it doesn't happen again, persuade yourself that the event or glitch was a weird onetime thing. Short-term memory loss (STML) is an inconvenience or a goddamn nuisance or an embarrassment—but it's *not* an illness. Consider this: for those with dementia, daily living activity is not possible without constant and comprehensive aid. If that's not you, then it's not you.

Will short-term memory get worse over time? It may or may not. If it does, use memory aids like lists and pop-up reminders on your cell phone. But don't think you're about to become demented (a hallmark of Alzheimer's).

Is there a medication that will help STML? None have been proven to do so, but the promise of taking a daily pill to eliminate STML sells products. I mean, the snake oil of some exotic animal may feel good when massaged into arthritic joints, but a memory treatment? Don't think so!

Do memory games or challenges help? I think so, but there is no hard and fast evidence. But doing crossword puzzles or sudoku or word games is fun and a sort of evidence that your intellect is functioning. Good for the ego! I've already mentioned that I am a competitive *Jeopardy!* player. No matter the score, I always enjoy it.

I must reiterate, short-term memory loss is very, very common as we age. But it's not a disease, nor is it an illness of any sort. So don't complain. Play brain-stimulating games for distraction and boasting rights. And start writing things down more on a notepad or phone app.

Fear is a miserable thing to live with, dread perhaps even more so. So don't let them crop up when they're absolutely uncalled for. The beginning of almost any physical ailment or condition may resemble many, many others, but then it may go no further. Few ailments develop into something medically severe or disabling. You need to watch for repeat occurrences or more severe symptoms. According to the Alzheimer's Association (www.alz.org), only about 10 percent of Americans over age sixty-five develop Alzheimer's.

Alzheimer's is a disease. Progressive, disabling, and untreatable, leading to early demise. The progress of the disease may be rapid (in which case, diagnosis is not a problem) or slow. But frequently, it involves far more serious health issues than memory failure. Alzheimer's might include an overall misperception of events along with small movement failures such as an inability to button small buttons. It can involve clumsiness with larger movements and balance. Brain scans are an early diagnostic for the disorder. And it is *not* caused by short-term memory loss.

One more time: short-term memory loss does not lead to dementia (Alzheimer's). No way, no how, and never!

Nodding Off

DR. H

When you're a young child, there is a designated nap time. The hours and location are immutable. And there are penalties if these parameters are transgressed!

As you reach your sixties, and especially when you've arrived beyond that number, you tend to nod off, sometimes at really inappropriate times (e.g., when visitors come in the afternoon or early evening, or even when someone is talking to or about you!).

These nod-offs can only be called unfortunate, but they can also be viewed as almost antisocial or maybe an embarrassment to your family.

My favorite uncle, Julien, was one of the brightest, most articulate, and with-it people I knew (certainly among my gang!) well into his nineties. But when he came to visit one afternoon, in the midst of having high tea and swapping recent family news, he began to nod off and drool slightly. Much as I loved and admired him, it was a physical put-off and reminder of his age and lessening faculties.

Personally, the thought of being caught nodding off on social occasions is horrifying. However, I find myself doing so at less-than-stirring theater performances. Did you really find *Hair* all that fascinating? I mean, *Phantom of the Opera* or *Chicago* will hold my attention, but *Miss Saigon*? Yes, boredom, or repetitive conversation, inclines Old Broads to nod off.

If anything can justify the world calling you someone to be pitied as *old*, it's this habit—these drop-off (actually, drop-out) moments in the middle of a conversation or activity. You're automatically out of the loop, and you can't create a regrouping or catch-up when you jolt awake.

You can and should do something drastic about inappropriate, right-in-the-middle-of-things napping or nodding off. If you don't take these senior nod-offs in hand, you may well be blackballed from ongoing events, conversations, and visits. No matter how much love you are surrounded by, these particular senior moments will not and should not be tolerated.

So, what can you do to avoid this?

What I did was recognize afternoon and early evening tendencies and try not to risk matters. I refused to visit during vulnerable hours. Being part of top management in our home, I had the power to do so. But you might think about one or more of these suggestions:

- Go back to childhood-designated nap times. Let the household know the scheduling, and be consistent.
- Schedule visits and activities during times when you can control nod-offs. For instance, in the first part of the morning or in the late afternoon (after a nap).
- Do your best to get adequate sleep at night. It does no good if you're bright and perky when the household has settled in for the night.

The solutions I propose are far from a foolproof system, but they're a start. Use your smarts to effectuate your own particular anti–nod off campaign. Go for it, and defeat anyone who may suggest you're not sufficiently and/or consistently "with it."

What should you do if you nod off and someone makes fun of you? Humph. I wouldn't suggest my way of handling this problem without the consent of your entire household, but in mine, these people have been asked to leave. That said, generally this type of age mockery isn't part of my social circle.

GETTING GOOD SLEEP

Now, sleep is really a different matter altogether. Inadequate sleep results in both physiological and psychological consequences. The physiological includes things such as easy fatigue, while the psychological may lead to ill-temper or impatience. I think you will be familiar with or even have experienced these. What you may not recognize is that lack of adequate sleep may also lead to inattention, which, in quick turn, can lead to harmful negative consequences—everything from a slip and fall to a burned or pricked finger. Or nodding off! All highly undesirable.

Your MD will tell you that four hours of uninterrupted sleep is a minimum requirement. If you're a poor sleeper, there are some tried-and-true aids:

- Read a book on a subject you always meant to cover—not a bodice ripper or murder mystery or anything that could induce wakefulness. It's okay if you don't remember what you read or only remember a small bit. It's also okay if your progress is markedly slow. If it's boring, it can be a sleep inducer.
- Talk to your MD about over-the-counter sleeping pills or natural aids to see what might be helpful for you.

- Count sheep (as the old idea goes) or deer or buffalo or whatever other four-footed creature you like. The effectiveness of this method is a matter of how you do it. The counting must be slow, soft, and uninterrupted by thoughts for it to work.
- Listen to soft, old-fashioned music or check out stations on the TV or phone apps that are designed to help you fall asleep.
- Finally, you may imagine yourself on a warm summer afternoon, gently swaying in a hammock asleep. In other words, picture a sleep-inducing image of yourself.

The jury is out on whether a short daytime nap interferes with your nighttime sleep. Part of the answer is trying to limit naps to no more than one hour. Either set an alarm or get a reliable person to wake you up so you stick with the schedule.

When you were young, you either just closed your eyes if you were the least bit drowsy or you were able to do that at an appropriate time. But as we enter our senior years, as it is with so many habits or activities, things typically change. What is of most importance is that you exert some control to make sleep as voluntary as possible and not an involuntary event.

To sum up, unlikely as it seems, naps may become a controversial subject and loom large domestically. Don't let that happen. Pick and choose your time.

WHOOPI'S TWO CENTS

I don't understand naps and sleep. Everybody says you need to get a whole bunch of sleep, but for some reason, naps are not for me. I don't like them. I always feel drugged when I wake up from a nap.

Maybe that's because I've been drugged. I don't know for sure. But I'm pretty sure that some people just can't nap.

I'm not a big napper, I'm not a big sleeper, but that's how I've always been, and if you've been like that most of your life, don't worry about it. Just do you.

An Approach to
Your Will

DR. H

When I turned twenty-one my trust wrote to me that I needed to make a will. Can you imagine? Right at what I considered to be the beginning of my adult life, here were these men—these financial men—saying I had to do something I associated with the end of life.

In truth, I did have some money. But again, at age twenty-one? A will?

I found out that if I had no kids to inherit, the money would go to the state. In short, if I were intestate, the state was not. I also learned, as I'm sure many of you know, that the signing of my will had to be witnessed. The thought of this solemn legal moment sent me into uneasy laughter. I mean, really old people conceded themselves with this kind of thing, but me?

Then I thought for a minute about the way I drove after hoisting any number of drinks. And yes, I shake my head at my younger self doing that way-beyond-stupid thing. But a will suddenly made sense.

Long story short, I did make a will, leaving most of my funds to the American Society for the Prevention of Cruelty to Animals.

Not a bad choice, but who you wish to benefit from your demise may alter over the years.

After I became an MD and saw too often what happened in city emergency rooms, I redrew and certified the will. So that was done when I was still at a young age, relatively speaking. Done and thought no more of. I still felt animals were more worthy than most other causes.

You can create a legal will as long as you have a legal testament, but that's not always the way to go. It may create room for disagreement or hardship. I find that, if asked, your attorney will refer you to an appropriate specialist to ensure that what you are doing is legal and will be carried out.

LIFE'S REALITY

There comes a day when you realize you must draw up a will that reflects your mature wishes for the inheritance of your possessions, whether a few sticks of furniture or a significant estate.

Almost nobody wants to face or deal with the matter of wills. They allude to the end of life, a thought that causes most of us to feel a degree of—let's call it what it is—fear. Fear of the unknown and un-when and un-how.

In essence, for most of us, the topic of wills seems to be unwelcome and is often put off as long as possible. It may also involve difficult decisions as to who and what.

Hold the fort! Katy bar the door! Let's talk Old Broad to Old Broad.

Making a will at this age isn't called an act of happiness, yet maybe it should be. Wouldn't you feel happy to know that you've arranged the memory you want others to have of you?

So straighten your spine and get out a large notepad. Start by collecting several photos of moments you've spent together with inheriting friends, children, and grandchildren. Get them framed if they aren't already. Remember the power of a visual prompt to bring to life a time or spot or association, and take pleasure in this visual collection. Next, find mementos you've shared. This may include personal favorite jewelry or favorite recipes—really anything you can think of that you wish to be remembered by. They are part of the inheritance.

I'm a believer in the written word (obviously). I think leaving words to be read by your near and dear on your demise is important, cogent, generous, and thoughtful. An inheritance even more valuable than the sticks of furniture. Whether you're Bill Gates or someone living off of food stamps, this gesture of love and caring is, as your grandkids might say, the most!

Write your loved ones words of affection or wisdom that are unique to you. If there's a meaningful book you've shared, inscribe a few words on the title page and make it a part of your will.

The reading of a will can be a cold and dreary experience for those in the room. Yes, you're required to deal with your possessions, but that part of things should be very much ameliorated by what we're trying to do here, which is to create a personal remembrance, Mama Bear to inheritor.

Hopefully, whatever you do with your estate, you choose to distribute things such as money, art, and houses in an equitable way—or in a way that does not stir negative thoughts or emotions between those you'll leave behind. To make this more meaningful, write a word or two about each bequest, accompanied by a personal memory.

I think you get my point. Making a will is a positive, lasting, and person-to-person event. Whoop will be remembered for her extraordinary movie characterizations and cybernetically for *The View*. Most of us don't have these public markers, but don't let the drawing up of a will become a "Woe is me" that brings a foretaste of your demise into what can be a moment of creative memory.

Let's Talk
About Attrition

DR. H

Hunter S. Thompson wrote, "Life should not be a journey to the grave with the intention of arriving safely in a pretty and well preserved body, but rather to skid in broadside in a cloud of smoke, thoroughly used up, totally worn out, and loudly proclaiming 'Wow! What a Ride!'"

Boy, was he right!

In my teens I swam regularly across the mountain waters of Lake Rangeley in Maine, just because I could. Mine was a swim of approximately one and a half miles in water that I considered warm at sixty-five degrees. At the age of fifty-five, I "dipped" three times a day in Lake Rangeley—meaning I took a quick swim of about a hundred yards out and back from the dock.

When you enter your later fifties, your physical appearance and function is unlikely to look or be the same as it may have once been. This is what is meant by attrition. You have little or no choice in the matter, so there's no point in grieving over it. Human physiology being human physiology, aging has this impact.

Fortunately, it is not an equally true indication of mental capacity or acuity, which may actually increase with seniority. Wisdom is the precise opposite of mental attrition. And there are different degrees of attrition from person to person.

Aches and pains come with the territory of age. Think about it! You have been using your bones, muscles, and tendons for these many years. Don't you think they may get tired as well? Typically, and most often, body aches originate with osteoarthritis (the wear-and-tear type of arthritis). Osteoarthritis involves the back, hips, knees, and, unfortunately, sometimes the hands and fingers. Our forebears used to call osteoarthritis "rheumatism," which is why today rheumatoid arthritis is so often confused with the more common form.

We begin to fear that attrition is going to progress rapidly as a kind of bodily visitation. This is a time to do your best to step aside or out of your body and make the assessment of what's going on, as if this were an evaluation by your best friend. It's tough, but you can't over- or underrate what's happened. Then, once you complete your evaluation, keep moving forward.

WAYS TO HELP
OR SLOW PROGRESSION

As a physician and a human being, I know some of the ways arthritis (a form of attrition) produces aches and pains and also leads to a diminution of range of motion, dexterity, and the strength to accomplish so many of life's daily activities. I think you will be familiar with much of what follows here, but I want to talk about something that is not always considered important.

Single or one-by-one treatments or medications can modify aches and pains to a degree, but combinations can be used to increase treatment efficacy. Even treatments that may seem like one-offs may be augmented by add-ons.

SURGERY, MEDICATION, AND PHYSICAL THERAPY

Surgery is the most radical treatment of arthritis affecting hips, knees, and shoulders. It consists of joint replacement, and before you say, "But not for me—I'm seventy, eighty, or ninety," not so fast! If your overall health is sound, you are a perfectly good candidate for surgical joint replacement. Many are done and done successfully for this older group. And the pre- and post-condition difference is, in a word, amazing!

Now let's talk briefly about medications, including anti-inflammatory medications (of which there are dozens available over the counter), which, if taken regularly, can modify aches and pains. This is especially true if they are combined with a gentle over-the-counter analgesic pain reliever. Your pharmacist can help you secure one of these.

Lastly, I don't want to forget physical therapy (PT). If it's taught and/or supervised by an experienced and qualified individual, I am a big believer in the benefits of legitimate PT.

But to get back to attrition: Your family, children, and/or grandchildren will encourage you to exercise with a capital E (denoting their concept or practice of exercise). All too often, this may be beyond your ability or competence. So try this: "Let me tell you about attrition." Most will look at you as if you've begun to talk Swahili. To which you can respond, "It's my attrition," and smile like the sly fox you are. Then offer your bicep and ask that they feel your muscle so expectations all around become more realistic.

Again with a fox-like smile, you may go on to say, "Attrition is the opposite of ripped." That is verbal game, set, and match! But if you're kind in victory, you can add, "Attrition, which is a part of living beyond twenty, deserves not necessarily respect but acknowledgment."

Breaking Medical News

DR. H

This is a truly difficult, tough, and even tricky issue facing all of us over sixty! But sharing your medical news with others is essential if you care about independence and having a generally enjoyable existence. However, the conversation must be carefully organized, planned, and monitored by you.

When it comes to any kind of conversation that deals with your health, life decisions, and overall well-being, I've developed these thoughts:

- *Set the agenda.* Ideally, it will have no more than two foci. If you try to cover more, you may find either that you wander or your family's attention is dispersed. Your presentation must be sharp, completely focused, and ready to address each discussion point.
- *Be prepared.* Be sure that your needs in light of these issues are clear, and be open to possible compromise. Also ensure the information you share is medically or scientifically well informed.

- *Stay cool.* Approach the talk as a business executive meeting with their board to get something done or initiated. Here, emotionality must, as far as possible, be eliminated. You want to be calm, practical, and logical.
- *Set ground rules.* Don't permit digression or an emotional reaction to destroy the program you've set. You may have to say, "Let's not wander from the issue," or "You raise an interesting point—hold on to it till we're finished with the matter we're discussing."
- *Ask yourself the what-ifs.* In your preplanning, try to guess what objections or questions may arise given what you know about your family.

When the time is right for you, simply request a meeting with your nearest and dearest—either in person, over the phone, or using a computer app like Zoom or FaceTime—without any indication of subject. You don't want to catch anyone off guard, so keep the request simple, telling them you would like their input on an important matter.

I had a dear friend who needed a pacemaker. She knew her family and close friends would be upset with the news. Since everyone was not local to discuss this in person, my friend decided to craft an email to break the news (have the family discussion online) and alleviate any additional concerns. Her note spoke of the problem, the solution, and the outcome. Here's what she wrote:

Hi, all,

For many of you, this may be the first time you are hearing of my health issue with my heart—the past few weeks have certainly been a *big* surprise—but I wanted to hold off on any updates until I had a clear path with a diagnosis and plans to move forward.

First, I want everyone to know that my prognosis is great—my surgeon says "way better" than great, so I am all for that!

How it all started: Visit to my GP for a sinus infection to get meds before a business trip. Normal checks: blood pressure—great; pulse oxygen—perfect; and then heart rate—the nurse asked, "Do you know your heart rate is only forty BPM?" (Normal resting heart rate is sixty to one hundred BPM.)

Next thing you know, I'm having an EKG. My heart rate is thirty-four BPM and in something called atrial flutter (sawtooth). I had been walking and talking—I'd even driven my car to the appointment (to the complete amazement of the docs). But there would be no more driving for me that day. They called an ambulance, and off I went to the ER.

Hospital Visit: Diagnosed with atrial flutter (when the heart's rhythm is out of sync. Some people have problems with the heart's "plumbing," while I have a problem with the heart's electrical or conduction system). Good news is that they can *cure* the atrial flutter with something called atrial ablation. So, on February 10, I had the atrial ablation procedure on my heart to cure the flutter and get my heart back into rhythm. The procedure worked, but the surgeon was planning for my heart rate to be back around seventy BPM, only to find out that it had a mind of its own and liked being closer to thirty BPM.

Enter "You have Wenckebach phenomenon": it's when pulses (electrical signals) from the top of the heart don't all get sent through to the bottom. Some of them get blocked—easiest way to put it, a heart-rhythm disturbance. (Wish it had a cooler name like "Superwoman phenomenon.") Come to find out Wenckebach is common in many highly trained athletes who have undergone high-endurance, high-intensity training. Going back, I have documented that, as early as my late twenties, my heart rate was around forty BPM. Never paid any attention.

The Path Forward—Pacemaker: After numerous weeks of tests with monitors, treadmills, and watching my heart rate daily, our go-forward plan is to get my heart rate back up where it belongs. The way to get everything where it needs to be is to install a pacemaker. It will only act as an assistant to my heart. When my heart rate goes too low it will kick it back up to where it needs to be.

I have an excellent surgeon. He said my life expectancy could be even longer with the pacemaker—so good to know that I can keep my Nike commercial for my hundredth birthday.

Lemonade: On April 14, the pacemaker will be installed, and the mystery will finally be answered that I am actually bionic. I will only be in the hospital for one night. I am ready to "go get it" and make some lemonade with this life experience. I have too many other adventures planned and will gladly check the box on this one as "been there, done that!"

I hope this covers everything. I can't thank you all enough for your love and support.

What you see from this letter to the family is how my friend set the agenda and established a calm, collected, and a bit funny tone. Most importantly, she focused on the positive outcome to put everyone at ease.

These conversations with your family can be tough and emotional, and they become trickier as we age. At best your family will want to accede to what makes you happiest. Your obligation is to make clear that you're capable of handling the new setup and that it may have advantages for them, too, if indeed that is the case.

I can think of numerous ways to resolve situations where the family says, "We don't want you to," when you want to. Take, for example, driving a car at an advanced age. You can either prepare for hostility and say, "It's my car, and I will be its driver," or take a more accommodating approach: "I have noticed some dings recently, so perhaps somebody should be my copilot." You could also offer to take a new driver's test, which should include a test of your vision. It's bending over backward, but if that's your relationship with your family, it certainly is a goody-two-shoes solution.

One counter element that may underlie a medical talk is the role reversal that may, to some extent, have taken place in your medical decision-making due to physical limitations, short-term memory problems, or the demands necessitated by a change in your health requirements. I don't know entirely how to deal with this possible role reversal other than to suggest that, if it happens, you should try to maintain your cool and your own "adulthood" as much as possible.

When you need to schedule a meeting to address broader household issues, try this: First and always, go into the scheduled meeting as its CEO. Open the meeting with the topics you want to talk about (no more than three per session). Then, listen to what your family wants and adjust your own wants to a reasonable degree.

These are only some ideas to help you through family discussions. There are many, many ways to go about them. You know the strengths and weaknesses of your proposals, and you also know the attitudes of most of your family members. Always remember that you can negotiate and try this approach: "That's a good thought. Let's hold on to it and come back a second time to visit when we've each had a chance to think over this conversation." After all, not everything in this world can be decided in one sitting.

So, armed for the fray and ready to disarm it, try for a good night's rest the day before the talk is scheduled.

Then go for it, my fellow Broad CEOs.

WHEN YOUR EXCRETIONS
OUTWEIGH YOUR SECRETIONS

When have you officially arrived at senior status? There have been many definitions, either numeric, anecdotal, or statistical, that seek to define what it is to be an older citizen. The one I like best is this medical one: when your excretions outweigh your secretions.

Yes, that's a gag between wiseass MDs, but as with so many terse aphorisms, it's right on. As you've seen, telling it like it is has been my approach to medicine—even after retirement.

To make the observation clear if it is not already so, let me offer examples of each.

Secretions include sweat, for example as the by-product of a workout or lack of air-conditioning on a hot summer day. They also include the production of facilitating fluids during vigorous sexual contact.

Excretions include not-fully-controlled urination, also occasional defecation, or a constantly dripping nose.

I won't comment on the desirability of each, with the exception of the sexual connotation, as there is little choice in the matter. And I can't comment on their couth. What I will comment on is the need to enter senior status with a good sense of humor, personal hygiene and worth, and as much inventiveness as possible. These are all weapons to be evoked and called into battle.

Unfortunate, perhaps, but your status will be clear as glass if your excretions outweigh your secretions.

Crotchety with Charm

DR. H

Your simple technical or mechanical order arrives, but it's all wrong or it needs an encyclopedia, plus significant computer engineering guru skills to make it operational.

Someone bumps into you because they didn't bother to look and see you coming.

People smile to your face but diss you once your back is turned (someone always rats them out).

Or you just plain "get up on the wrong side of the bed."

You don't have to be Mrs. Nice Lady! Let it out! Express just what and how you feel about it—in as many four-letter words as you know.

It won't undo or fix the problem, but you'll feel a lot better about not playing Ms. Milquetoast. And you won't go to bed thinking of what you might have said. No way! 'Cause you've said it!

If this approach gives you pause, remember, as an Old Broad you can be legitimately crotchety as long as you coat it with charm when there's someone else in the room. ☺

PART SIX
Broad Insights

You have to believe in yourself in spite
of what other people believe.
WHOOPI GOLDBERG

———

LISTS ARE YOUR FRIENDS

A MORNING PRAYER

WHO ARE YOU CALLING ECCENTRIC?

THE SUNDAY COMICS

GROW OLD OR GROW UP?

BATTLE HYMN OF THE REPUBLIC

AN EVENING PRAYER

VALE DICTA (LAST WORDS)

BROAD ENCORE

Lists Are Your Friends

DR. H

This is a shortie, but I hope it's full of wisdom that makes you exclaim, "Oh my goodness, that's right!"

Lists are your friend! What you've written down, or entered on your iPhone, is your unvarying counter to short-term memory loss. You'll never lose anything because you've captured it in an L-I-S-T! Doing so makes you both smart and independent.

There's a secondary satisfaction to be gained by a long list, most especially if it's a list of things you need to do: you get to cross things off as they're accomplished. Done! *Finito!*

In general, consistency is a must. If you leave an article or item in the same spot consistently, you'll know, night or day, rain or shine, Monday or Thursday or any other day, where the item lives. It's a matter of logic—giving everything its own place, both on a list and when it comes to the list itself.

Also, repetition is a first cousin to consistency. Repetition can help when used as a memory aid, but it can become annoying, both to yourself and others, if employed too often. By repetition alone, some things will stay mentally current, fixed, and available for you when you need them.

Incidentally, repetition may also become a permanent visitor in the way you live if your sleeping, eating, and general activities tend to recur every day at a certain time. This may not entirely suit you (particularly those of us who don't take well to regimentation), but if caretakers are involved, repetition becomes an unarguable fact of life. You may discuss varying things, but in the end, you usually have to accede to routine. Do it with all the grace you can muster.

I started with lists but had to go to these other thoughts on the grounds that short-term memory loss needs all the counters we can give it. So now we have it: an armamentarium of protective concepts to subvert short-term memory loss!

WHOOPI'S TWO CENTS

Nobody should have the ability to talk you into anything that you don't want to do because you've earned the right to be the person you want to be. You've earned the right to have some fun at your age. But you've gotta take care of yourself.

And you know what else you've got to do? You've got to make lists. When in doubt, write it down. I know, I know, you think you're old—you are. Write it down.

Save yourself the strum and horror of trying to remember stuff. Keep pencils and pads everywhere. I don't care what they say on television, there's no pill for this. Get yourself together. Write it down because you'll feel much better. You can do this.

A Morning Prayer

DR. H

Let me remember to listen to a fall of rain or watch for the radiance of dawn.

Let me remember the miracle of a garden, where a small, desiccated seedling becomes a head of verdant lettuce or the green cup of a deep-purple eggplant

And savor the odors and taste of the kitchen.

Let me remember to listen for birds as they wing thru the sky and bless the familiarity of their song.

Let me wonder at the munificence of the planet Earth, my home

And the eternity of the cosmos it inhabits

And ask to save the least-deserving of its creatures: mankind.

Who Are You Calling Eccentric?

DR. H

My beloved grandmama Stein (née Hecht) was born in San Francisco, one of four sisters, each of whom was known for a particular trait. Grandmama was the youngest and was able all her life to charm the most diverse groups of people with ease, no matter their age, persuasion, or oddity. Then came my great-aunt Sally, who was known as a beauty from the time she was a young woman and all the way into her senior years. My aunt Hilda was a superb linguist, speaking as a native in four languages and conversant in twenty others.

My aunt Grace, the eldest, was a gourmet cook with an unrelenting sweet tooth. For her, all food led to dessert. She checked out all dessert creations the day before they were to be served at luncheons and dinners.

On April 18, 1906, Aunt Grace knew that she was to enjoy one of her particular and rarely done favorites: a blancmange, an angel-light pudding, created from a whipped cream, whipped egg white, and spun sugar. As I was later informed, a melt-in-your-mouth

French creation. It's no longer seen on dessert lists, except perhaps in a few traditional restaurants in Paris. But then it was the hall-mark of a supreme gourmet dessert.

On the afternoon of April 18, the now-infamous San Francisco earthquake destroyed far more than her dessert. Her entire house-hold's activities, aside from necessary cooking, ceased for the next five weeks.

Aunt Grace came to Baltimore in the mid-1930s for a visit with our extended family. I had just turned eight and was thus permit-ted a seat at the grown-up table during her welcoming luncheon, along with a dozen or so others.

The beginning course included plates of Chesapeake Bay oys-ters. As each set was placed, no one commented when Robert the butler placed a large slice of angel food cake, draped in whipped cream and confectioners' sugar, in front of my aunt Grace.

I had just enough couth not to stare and not to question. But I was absolutely consumed with curiosity. (Under similar circum-stances, wouldn't you have been too?)

Later that afternoon, after Grandmama's postprandial nap and a session doing braille for the blind, which she did every day, I went to see her.

She looked up before I said a word and said, "Mary Ellen, con-sider the consequences of that awful earthquake day in San Fran-cisco. From April 18, 1906, to the present, no matter where she dines, Aunt Grace has vowed never again to be caught without dessert. To make sure this doesn't happen, she starts every meal with dessert. Can you find any flaw with her reasoning?"

People referred to Aunt Grace as "eccentric." But was she? Or was hers a fine observation followed by irrefutable logic?

As I've started to think about the meaning of the word *eccen-tric*, I've realized there are many different synonyms in current use: oddball, once in a lifetime, far out, and just short of loony.

To me, they don't capture the sharply caught undertone of the word *eccentric*.

Sure, there were those who thought Aunt Grace was pixelated. But many more understood the aptness of her behavior. How many of us get to defy an earthquake?

Perhaps it is time to rescue eccentricity from the fastness of "strange" and place it where it may well belong: among the personally courageous and finely defining.

To be different or eccentric is to make plain your individuality, or why you can't be classified into a neat generality. Someone wrote a brilliant and apt description. You march to the cadence of the drummer's beat you hear.

The Sunday Comics

DR. H

Did you get too sophisticated, or did you always yearn for Sunday to come, when all your favorite comic characters appeared in riotous color?

In our house my younger sister and I beat the adults to the newspaper on Sundays to extract the comic section. Then we'd get our weekly fix of *The Katzenjammer Kids, Little Orphan Annie, Dick Tracy, Popeye, Terry and the Pirates, Bringing Up Father,* and *Toonerville Folks,* to mention only a few.

After we had each read our favorites balloon to balloon and gone in turn to the less-preferred characters, we were far from through. On the grounds that even the adults should share the fantastic experience, we sat down and carefully prepared a "movie of the week" for them.

We cut out our favorites into horizontal strips, then pasted them together with flour and water to create a continuous strip.

Our "screen" consisted of a box used to deliver clothes into which we had cut a six-inch by six-inch opening.

After the adults were suitably seated, we placed ourselves on either side of the box. Then we kneeled at either end of the box and ran the pasted strips through the screen with suitable narration based on the cartoon balloons.

When finished, either due to a major break in the pasted strip or having completed our movie without mishap, the adults applauded, and we each took our bows.

Kids today still get a comics section in the Sunday newspaper, but the topics are more involved with AI or sci-fi creatures—their action more explosive than personal.

The audience to whom we showed our movies has long gone, as have most of the comics from the '30s, and the artists who created and drew those beloved characters are no longer with us. I don't know about you, but the regularity with which favorite comic characters came in the Sunday papers was a part of childhood I'd thought would never change. Since then, the world has changed.

But if you want a whiff of your childhood every once in a while, you can still find some of the old comic characters' adventures in Big Little Book collections. These can be found in small second-hand bookstores or perhaps in the new "big little book"—online.

Grow Old or Grow Up?

DR. H

Virtually all of us Old Broads, newly hatched or well into the ages, have a basic, no—an unavoidable—choice. In so many words, a fight to be fought and won every day.

As Old Broads, our choice is this: maintain the keenness of our age-proven, hard-won thinking and perceiving abilities or get lazy, even sloppy, and make excuses—especially to ourselves. The latter leads to a C-minus or D-plus type of existence. *Yech!*

I turned ninety-two in the middle of editing this book, so I've learned a thing or two about time. I suppose I might have anticipated a long life—after all, my mother graced this world for 102 years. I've lost a lot of my friends—not from age but due to their *aging*. They grew old and away from me, from longtime friends, from society, and even from their families. This is a chapter I hope you read slowly, and don't let it put your back up.

Our goal in writing this book was to help make aging easier, amenable, and more understandable—but reality is also reality. Assuming you are not physically overwhelmed by arthritic, pulmonary, cardiac, or kidney problems—that is, you're able to dominate the character of your life with your mind and not become overwhelmed with pain or disability—ask yourself the following questions:

- Are you willing to grow less and less important in your family constellation, especially whenever important topics come up?
- Are you content to accept more and more passivity and willing to receive whatever is offered to you, whether it fits your needs and desires or not?
- Do you feel more and more disconnected from the life around you?
- Are you starting to feel more passive and "out of the moment"?

If none of those questions describes you, move on to the next chapter.

But if you answered yes to any of those questions, please consider long and hard the observations underlying my advice here. You want to make sure you're not permitting yourself to "grow old." Any one of the descriptions above can happen gradually or subtly. You have to guard against their occurrence almost before they occur.

The first or second time you find yourself accepting something either physically, socially, or mentally that is not right or necessary for you, the battle must begin. And, in a very real sense, end.

Don't get me wrong; I'm not suggesting rebellion or argumentation. But I do recommend opposition. Break out the charm if you prefer that route. But be sure your input in opposition counts.

Of course, there are times when going with the flow can work to your benefit. My caveat is you must remember what constitutes *your benefit* rather than what may be easy for somebody else or defined by them.

"Do not go gentle into that good night," as Dylan Thomas wrote. Demand the most of yourself. Prevent or obviate passivity and its accompanying need to take only what others propose. It's up to you to remain a contributing member of the clan and let people know you're a part of current society.

Make an effort to spot a problem, however minor, and come up with a solution before someone else in the family does. Both you and they will see what I mean by growing up rather than growing old. And remember, your active participation in the world is as good for your family as it is for you.

Personally, I'm both a busybody and a wisenheimer. I pick up hot-button topics from the discussions around me, then do internet research or find armamentarium from my days in theater or medicine or from my travels or academia. Then I come armed, whether invited or occasionally uninvited, to the fray.

Never think because your idea may be "out of fashion" that it's invalid or invaluable. You have years of living, experiencing, succeeding, and, yes, failing. Intellectual flexibility is what's required. And this exercise, like physical ones, is very good for your "core" mental being.

If you are able to come up with enough ideas about or answers to controversial subjects or happenings, you have the golden opportunity of becoming the "great compromiser" of your household. This enables you to become more and more integral, even when it comes to minor and major conundrums.

Remember, Broads, you can become the wise woman of your tribe. Your choice. (Big drumroll!)

Battle Hymn of the Republic

DR. H

The first line of this stirring hymn reads, "Mine eyes have seen the glory of . . ."! Which is why I've titled this chapter, written for caretakers or aides who support our elder citizens, after the "Battle Hymn of the Republic." Old Broads are valuable! And as you care for them, you need to remember:

- Never equate physical frailty with a lack of mental acuity and intuitiveness.
- Knees may stop their normal function; never consider the knee a part of the brain.
- A lack of acute hearing does not mean a lack of keenness. It means difficulty *hearing*.
- An Old Broad's eyes and ears have seen and heard much that yours haven't, so open your ears and eyes to their wisdom. You may be astonished by the depth and breadth of the experience.

- Some degree of short-term memory loss doesn't negate your favorite Old Broad's wealth of perception. Those many long years of memory can produce astonishing material. You and your Old Broad may get a surprising kick out of its contents if both of you take the time and trouble to talk and listen.
- If you're, let's say, in your thirties, forties, or fifties, these few years between you and an Old Broad don't entitle you to ignore her. Sometimes a lack of years suggests lack of perception.
- An approach of, "stop, look, and listen" might render you to an invaluable reward.
- There's a hell of a difference between being a caretaker (hired or volunteer) and being a helpful figure who is truly best called a caregiver. Does this difference strike home?

Just remember that those senior eyes may well have looked and seen many things. Upon them, glory.

WHOOPI'S TWO CENTS

———

Hey, God! You better let me wake up tomorrow! You hear?

An Evening Prayer

DR. H

I think most of us have a few moments before we go to sleep, and in these moments, we often review the day that has passed. I would like to suggest some thoughts to be included during this time that could come under the heading of remembering a day before abandoning it for night.

Let me take advantage of the things I'm good at but minimize frustration at those I'm not.

Let me conquer short-term memory loss with the practical means of using lists.

Let me convince those who care for me that there are many things I can do safely, without help.

Let me remember and celebrate my experience and wisdom purchased at the price of age.

Let me try the new, assuming it is interesting and physically within my ability.

Let me share my knowledge with my near and dear in quiet moments.

And last, I suppose, let me wake to the new day.

And so, lay down to sleep.

WHOOPI'S TWO CENTS

———

Please, God, let me wake up tomorrow. Amen.

Vale Dicta
(Last Words)

DR. H

We hear over and over again these days that sixty is the new forty. An occasion of joy! Let the good times roll! It's meant as an expression observing the actuarial estimates that put life expectancy higher than ever before. Hip hip hooray!

Multibillion-dollar women's cosmetic companies are built on this perception that we can look forty at sixty. (Heaven help us, Broads!)

From age sixty on, life may not hold the promise that you like. It is often a matter of compromise: physically, financially, socially—but that does not give you, and never should give you, an excuse to sit out your life. If push comes to shove, you may be able to bring something brand new into your life—and the lives of others.

In other words, your experience may lead you to something new and different and not only encouraging but admirable.

So, does forty (plus a bit) bring the good times inferred by life expectancy figures? No! I think not if you're a realist, unseduced by deceptive slogans, products that don't perform as advertised, and perhaps growing inflation figures timed just as you arrive at a fixed income. I say the promise of forty is, more often than not, unfulfilled by reality. Remember the unimaginable speed with which things happen in present times.

But when it comes to the truth versus the myths of being an Old Broad, let's celebrate sixty, including the smarts gained, the enjoyment of previously overlooked small and large things, the increased perception and understanding of many of life's phenomena, and the friendships that have endured the years.

Let's treat sixty as sixty and be proud of it!

Broad Encore

DR. H AND WHOOPI

Here's to us, Broads! We're role models. Moms. Sisters. Aunts. Wise owls and rule breakers.

We have earned our stripes and acquired our wisdom from scratch because today, no convention is sacred, and our status is far from quo. This is what happens at sixty and beyond to doctors, comedians, artists, engineers, politicians, writers, homemakers, teachers, photographers, and everyone in between.

The world is littered with "could haves," "should haves," and "if onlys."

As proud Broads, we believe in "why nots"—the lives that present themselves every day, full of possibilities that leave us hoping we are better for having met them.

We do not believe in granny time, and we do not hide behind our Broadness. We are brave and brassy and just damn brilliant.

You have been unleashed—enjoy!

We're so glad we had this time together!

Epilogue

IN MEMORY OF M. E. HECHT, MD

DIANE SMITH

———

This book was Dr. M. E. Hecht's dream. She was excited to write it with her friend Whoopi and share her ninety-three years of wisdom with all Broads and the world. Dr. H passed away a few short months prior to publishing. As *the* quintessential Broad herself, she would be cheering all of you on.

Dr. H was the kind of person to make you think . . . a lot. She was interesting and interested in many things. She has been a continuous, vibrant, extraordinary thread running throughout my life and the lives of so many others. All of us and now countless new Broads have become part of the Dr. H tapestry.

And oh, what a beautiful tapestry Dr. H was—one full of authenticity, great intelligence, and color!

But, as with a tapestry, she would want all of us to understand that if one thread ends, we tie it off as best we can. No matter how difficult, we build off that thread and add new strands. The tapestry patterns will change a little or a lot, but we never forget that original thread and its beautiful color; we hold on to its deep teachings and share those teachings with others.

So here's to Dr. Mary Ellen Hecht. Dr. H to you. M'Ellen, M, and bud to me. Someone who dreamed big dreams and blazed new paths. Thank you for your personality, imagination, commitment, and love. You always told me that small stories never stir the soul—so go explore, challenge, and be visible in the world so it can find you.

Well, today the world has found *you*, Dr. H. I couldn't be more proud.

Dianne Smith is Dr. H's close friend and business partner.

WHOOPI

Mary Ellen and I met at a Ralph Rucci fashion show. I'm not sure how it came about, but next thing we knew, we were hanging out. There are so many stories I could tell you about what she thought we as humans could do better for our own edification, or our conversations about our different paths, but I won't because it's in this book. What you see is us really in conversation. I will also tell you she gave the best advice on being a human being. She believed in the fun of getting older and always wanted to make sure that you understood getting older was not for sissies.

She was funny and thoughtful, and she was someone who enjoyed life and lived it. Heed what she's written 'cause she's telling the truth.

I'm so glad I got to make her laugh and that she allowed me to chime in on her book. Make no mistake: she was a really funny woman, a really fine thinker, and . . . my friend.

Sail on, Silver Girl.

Acknowledgments

To my editor, Tamela: thank you for expanding my voice. Always wishing you a good morning. And to Andrea and the Harper Horizon team: I thank you for your unwavering support and confidence.

—DR. H

Index

A

"Ac-Cent-Tchu-Ate the Positive"
      (song), 10
accident avoidance, 135–38
aches and pains, 63–64
acuity, mental, 201
ADA (American Diabetes
      Association), 67
advice, parental, 19–20
aerobic exercise, 94, 128
age, as more than a number, 5–7
aging, 197–99
allergies, 147
Altman, 34
Alzheimer's disease, 159–61
American Diabetes Association
      (ADA), 67
American Society for the Prevention
      of Cruelty to Animals (ASPCA),
      169
amputation, with whiskey anesthesia,
      89
anesthesia, 89–90
ankle exercise, 120
anti-inflammatory medications, 95,
      113, 175
appearance, physical, 173
arthritis, 35, 45, 64, 94–95, 113,
      117–18, 174

ASPCA (American Society for the
      Prevention of Cruelty to
      Animals), 169
atrial ablation, 179
atrial flutter, 179
attrition, 173–76
audiologists, 99
automobile analogy, for human
      body, 11–13

B

Baker, Josephine, 3
ballroom dancing, 94
Baltimore, Md., xiv, 29, 53
bathing suits, 55–56
bedside manners, 74
Beene, Geoffrey, 34
Big Little Books, 196
bleeding, postoperative, 91
blind people, 97
bodies, human, 11–13, 16
bone fractures, 135
book clubs, 42
bores, 114
Botox, 124
bowling, 130
boxing, 130
breast self-examinations, 151–55
breathing exercise, 118

Bringing Up Father, 195
broad experience, 3–4
Broadway, xv, 33, 58
Bruce, Nigel, xiv
Bryn Mawr, Pennsylvania, xiv
bunion surgery, 49–50
bursitis, 64

C
Cabrini Medical Center, 139
calluses, 51
cancer, 125, 152, 154
cardiorespiratory exercise, 94
caretakers, 109, 201
CCC (Civilian Conservation Corps),
    102
Chicago (musical), 164
childproof medication containers,
    150
chiropodists, 50
choice, personal, 111
Civilian Conservation Corps (CCC),
    102
Cleveland Clinic, 67
climate change, 22
clothing, 33–35, 111. *see also footwear;*
    names of specific garments
cochlear implants, 99
Codeine, 148–49
Cohen, Alex, xv
comics, 195–96
common interests, 31
consistency, 187–88
conversations, one-to-one, 6–7
COVID-19 pandemic, xvi–xvii, 37,
    59, 125
Crosby, Bing, 10
crossword puzzles, 6, 99, 160
current events, 7, 110, 114, 134

D
dancing, ballroom, 94

dating, 37–43
dating services, 41
daytime sex, 46
dementia, 159–61
dentistry, 103–5
Dick Tracy, 195
diet, 105–6
diseases, sexually transmitted, 46
disinformation, medical, 68
doctor-patient relationship, 72
doctor's appointments, 146
dog parks, 42
dress, 33–35, 111
driving, 180–81
Drugs.com, 67
Dust Bowl, 21

E
ear, nose and throat specialists
    (ENTs), 99
eccentricity, 191–93
The Economist, 59
education, patient, 65–66
eHarmony, 41
Elle, 34
ENTs (ear, nose and throat
    specialists), 99
Evans, Madge, xiv
excursions, 57–60
exercise(s)
    aerobic, 94, 128
    bed, 118–22
    buddy, 132
    inactivity, vs., 113, 115
    morning, 117–22
    postoperative, 92–95
    see also specific forms of exercise
experience, 3–4, 21–22

F
fabrics, 124
FaceTime, 60, 178

Index

facial hair, 124
falls, 49–50, 139–41
family discussions, 177–82
FamilyDoctor.org, 67
farmers markets, 27
fashion, 33–35
fear of missing out (FOMO), 58
field trips, 58
fitness centers, 131
flexibility exercises, 93–94
FOMO (fear of missing out), 58
food, 17
foot massage, 51
footwear, 49–52, 111, 127–32
foreplay, 47
Four Ears, One Notepad, 67, 69–70,
   145
fractures, bone, 135
frailty, 201
Franklin, Aretha, xiii
friendships, 25–31, 29–31

G

games, brain-stimulating, 6, 99, 114,
   160, 161
general conditioning, 128
Gibson, Althea, 10
Ginsburg, Ruth Bader, 3
girdles, 53–55
gloves, 124
Goldberg, Whoopi, xiii, xv, 171–72
golf, 127, 129–30
Gone with the Wind (movie), 53
Grace, Aunt, 191–92
Grand Canyon, 60
group outings, 42
Guerlain, 46
gum treatment, 104, 106

H

Hair (musical), 59
hair, facial, 124

hammertoe surgery, 49–50
health care
   dental care, 101–6
   doctors appointments, 69–75
   patients as partners, 65–68
   second opinions, 81–84
hearing aids, 7, 99
hearing impairment, 97–99, 201
Hecht, M. E., xiv–xv
Hecht Group, 69
heels, 50, 51
helpers, 109–12
Hepburn, Katharine, 3
High Society (movie), 10
Hilda, Aunt, 191
history, 21–22
honeybee population, 22
horizons, broadening of, 27
humor, 134
hyaluronic acid, 124
hydration, of skin, 123–24

I

ikebana, 6
implants, dental, 104
inactivity, 113–15
independence, 109–12
infection, postoperative, 91
inhibitions, 115
insurance, medical, 80
interests, 7, 17
isolation, 97, 99

J

James, Charles, 55
Jeopardy!, 6, 159–61
Jimmy Choo (shoes), 49, 52
joint replacement, 86, 94, 117–18,
   175
jokes, 114
Julius Caesar, 35
JUVÉDERM, 124

K

Kama Sutra, 47
Kelly, Grace, 10
Kings County Hospital Center, 97
knees, 201
knitting, 6

L

LaCroix, Christian, 55
Lake Rangeley (Maine), 173
learning, continuous, 58
Lebowitz, Fran, 26
leg exercise, 120
Leigh, Vivien, 53
l'heure bleu, 46
Lillie, Bea, xiv
listening, passive, 114
lists, 187–88
Little Orphan Annie, 195
living in the past, 133–34
Louboutin (shoes), 52
Louvre, 60

M

malignancy, early signs of, 125
malnutrition, 105–6
mammograms, 154
Manolo Blahnik (shoes), 49
masking, xvi–xvii
masturbation, mutual, 47
Match, 41
Mayo Clinic, 67
McDaniel, Hattie, 53
Medicaid, 78
medical advice, 65–68
medical history, 69
medical news, sharing with others,
    177–82
Medicare and Medicaid, 78, 83
medication(s)
    anti-inflammatory, 95, 113, 175
    containers, 144, 150

list, 69
    reactions to, 146–47
    side effects of, 143, 145, 149
MedlinePlus, 67
meeting of Whoopi and Dr. Hecht,
    25–27
memory
    aids, 187–88
    loss, 159–61
    short-term, 17, 202
menstruation, 152
Merman, ethel, 81
Metropolitan Museum of Art, 60
missionary position, 45
Miss Saigon (musical), 164
mobility, 111
Mother Cabrini Hospital, xv
muscle-building exercises, 94
muscles, 113
musculoskeletal system, 117–22

N

napping, 163–65
National Institutes of Health (NIH),
    67
nausea, 143
neck exercise, 120
negativity, 9
neighborhood events, 42
news, keeping up with, 7, 110, 114,
    134
New York City, xiv, 33–34
New York Fashion Week, 25
New York University, xiv
Nicklaus, Jack, 127
NIH (National Institutes of Health),
    67
NoHo (New York City), 57–58
notepads, 17
novocaine, 103
nutrition and teeth, 105–6

O

Obama, Michelle, 3
obesity, 105, 152
online tours, 60
operas, 58
opiates, 148–49
orthopedic surgeons, 50
orthopedic surgery, xv
osteoarthritis, 174–75

P

pacemakers, 178, 180
pain, postoperative, 92
pain relievers, 175
Palmer, Arnold, 127
pantyhose, 54
parental advice, 19–20
Parks, Rosa, 3
patient education, 65–66
Pavarotti, Luciano, 59
peloton cycling, 129
perception, 202
Perle, Dr., 139–40
personal introductions, 42
pesticides, 22
Phantom of the Opera, 164
pharmacies, 148
phobia, dental, 101–6
physical activity, 127–32
physical therapists, 95
physical therapy, 175
physiology, human, 173–76
pigmentation, changes in, 125
pill containers, 144
pneumonia, double, 83
podiatrists, 50
Popeye, 195
Posen, Zac, 55
postcoronary patients, 45
postoperative complications, 91
prayer, 189, 203–4
prostate cancer, 154

puzzles and games, 114

R

range of motion exercise, 128
reactions to medications, 146–47
rehabilitation, postoperative, 91–95
repetition, 187–88
Rigoletto (opera), 59
robots, 43
role reversals in decision-making,
    181
Romero, Cesar, xiv
Roosevelt, Franklin Delano, 102
rowing machines, 129
rubber, 54
Rucci, Ralph, 25–26
running, 94

S

Saks Fifth Avenue, 34
Sally, Aunt, 191
San Francisco earthquake, 192
Savannah, Ga., xiv
Scarlett O'Hara (fictional character),
    53
schedules, 15–17
self-expression, 183
selflessness, 134
sepsis, 83
sex, 45–48
shampoos, 124
Shipley School, xiv, 29–30
shoes, 49–52, 111, 127–32
short-term memory, 159–61
shoulder exercise, 119
side effects of medications, 143, 145,
    149
SilverSingles, 41
Simpson, Adele, 34
Sinatra, Frank, 10
sitting up in bed, 120
skin care, 123–25

sleep, 165–67
sleeping aids, 165
Smith, Diane, 27, 31
soaps, 124
social activity, 114
social connections, 58
Social Security, 102
socks, 51
SoHo (New York City), 57–58
spandex, 54
speaker function of mobile phones, 99
spine, 45–46
spine exercise, 119
spinning, 129
sports footwear, 52, 127–32
Stein, Grandmama, 191
Stewart, Martha, 26
stimulation, sexual, 47
stop, look and listen, 136, 202
stretching, 115
sudoku, 6, 99, 160
Sullivan, Ed, 10
Sunday comics, 195–96
supplements, 149
surgery
    fear of, 77–80
    foot, 49–50
    joint replacement, 86, 94, 117–18, 175
    orthopedic, xv
    patients choosing surgeons, 87–88
    postoperative period, 91–95
    surgeons choosing patients, 85–87
    unnecessary, 79–80
swimming, 94, 127, 128
swimsuits, 55–56

T
Tailored Woman, 34
Talley, André Leon, 26
teeth, 101–6

teledildonics, 47
telemedicine, 150
telephones, hearing-enhanced, 99
tennis, 129
Terry and the Pirates, 195
theater, 35
Theater Guild, 33
Thomas, Dylan, 199
Thompson, Hunter S., 173
Three-Look Method, 136–37, 139, 202
time, 15–18
toes, 51
toning exercises, 94, 128
Toonerville Folks, 195
tours, online, 60
travel, 57–60
Trigère, Pauline, 34
TYLENOL, 95, 148–49

U
US Army Quartermaster Corps, xiv

V
Vanderbilt, Gloria, xiv
Versace, Gianni, 55
The View (TV show), 33, 172
vitamins and minerals, 149
Vogue, 26, 34
von Doz, Lucienne, 26

W
walkerettes, 111
walking
    barefoot, 51
    fast, 127, 130
water, in skin, 123–24
water aerobics, 94
WebMD, 67
weight lifting, 131
well-being, 109–55
    accident avoidance, 135–38

breast self-examinations, 151–55
falls, 49–50, 139–41
inactivity, 113–15
independence, 109–12
living in the past, 133–34
medications, 67, 69, 95, 113, 143–50, 175
morning exercises, 117–22
physical activity, 127–32
skin care, 123–25
Wenckebach phenomenon, 179
West, Mae, 3, 48
Wheel of Foreplay, 47

wills, 169–72
wisdom, 19–20, 201, 207
Women's Wear Daily, 34
World War II, 54
WPA (Works Progress Administration), 102

Y
Yale University, xv
yoga, 129

Z
Zoom, 37–38, 59, 178

About the Authors

M. E. Hecht, MD, was a renowned surgeon who brought innovation and healing to the world. A published author, freelance writer, and orthopedic surgeon, Dr. Hecht was a recognized expert with degrees from Yale, Columbia University, and the State University of New York, in addition to advanced study she undertook in Davos, Switzerland. After receiving her medical degree, Dr. Hecht became the assistant chief of orthopedics at Elmhurst Hospital, an affiliate of Mount Sinai School of Medicine. Always a brave innovator, she created the first ambulatory care unit for Cabrini Hospital and later established the country's first group of surgeons devoted solely to rendering second opinions for elective surgery, the Hecht Group Second Surgical Opinion Institution.

Dr. Hecht continued to present, write, and contribute as a medical expert to a variety of international publications on strength, exploration, care, and aging. Her philanthropic endeavors continue to abound, including her support for young artists by cofounding the Singers Development Foundation. She believed in growing older; growing "into it" but never "out of it." Her promise to do no harm was her life-guiding mantra.

Whoopi Goldberg is the bestselling author of *Is It Just Me?*, *If Someone Says "You Complete Me," Run!*, and *The Unqualified Hostess*, as well as her children's books, including *Alice, Whoopi's Big Book of Manners,* and the *Sugar Plum Ballerinas* series. She is a prolific producer and entrepreneur, and is one of a very elite group of artists who have won the Grammy, the Academy Award, the Golden Globe, the Emmy, and a Tony Award for her film, television, recording, and stage work.